Coping with Early

Jill Eckersley is a freelance writer with many years' experience of writing on health topics. She is a regular contributor to women's and general-interest magazines, including *Women's Running*, *Women's Fitness*, *Slimming World* and other titles. *Coping with Childhood Asthma*, *Coping with Childhood Allergies*, *Helping Children Cope with Anxiety*, *Every Woman's Guide to Heart Health*, *Living with Eczema*, *Every Woman's Guide to Digestive Health*, *Coping When Your Child Has Cerebral Palsy*, *Coping with Snoring and Sleep Apnoea* and *Coping with Dyspraxia*, nine books written by Jill for Sheldon Press, were all published between 2003 and 2010. She lives beside the Regent's Canal in north London with her cat.

Overcoming Common Problems Series

Selected titles

A full list of titles is available from Sheldon Press,
36 Causton Street, London SW1P 4ST and on our website at
www.sheldonpress.co.uk

Overcoming Common Problems Series

Overcoming Common Problems Series

Overcoming Common Problems

Coping with Early-onset Dementia

JILL ECKERSLEY

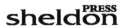
sheldon **PRESS**

First published in Great Britain in 2011

Sheldon Press
36 Causton Street
London SW1P 4ST
www.sheldonpress.co.uk

British Library Cataloguing-in-Publication Data
A catalogue record for this book is available from the British Library

ISBN 978-1-84709-130-7

1 3 5 7 9 10 8 6 4 2

Typeset by Fakenham Photosetting Ltd, Fakenham, Norfolk
Printed in Great Britain by Ashford Colour Press

Produced on paper from sustainable forests

Contents

Acknowledgements and note to the reader

Acknowledgements

I would not have been able to write this book without the help of many health professionals, and others, all of whom were unfailingly generous with their time and expertise. I would especially like to thank Kate Moffatt of the Alzheimer's Society, Tessa Gutteridge of the Clive Project, and Carol Jennings of the Pick's Disease Support Group. Carol kindly invited me to the group's London conference where I was able to benefit from hearing from clinicians, care-givers and those at the cutting edge of research into these cruel diseases.

Very special thanks are due to those people actually living with early-onset dementia, either as those with dementias or carers and family. Many spoke openly and frankly to me about the difficulties they face and the humour and love which have made the difficulties bearable. I hope I have done justice to your stories. Thank you all.

Note to the reader

This is not a medical book and is not intended to replace advice from your doctor. Consult your pharmacist or doctor if you believe you have any of the symptoms described, and if you think you might need medical help.

Introduction

Dementia is the catch-all term we usually use to describe a range of brain disorders which lead eventually to a complete loss of memory, speech, recognition and understanding. The most common form, Alzheimer's disease, is named after the German psychiatrist and neuropathologist who identified it in 1906. Alzheimer's is usually associated with older people and may affect as many as one in five of the over-85s. Dementia has been described as 'the greatest medical challenge of our time' as, with an ageing population, more and more people are likely to be affected, with all the implications that has for health and social care in the future.

However, dementia is not *just* a problem for the very old. Accurate figures are difficult to come by, but it is estimated that between 15,000 and 64,000 younger people – that is, people under 65 – in the UK have some form of dementia. About one-third of these are said to have Alzheimer's. It's difficult to say exactly how many because early-onset dementia, as it's known, can often be confused with other conditions and is sometimes misdiagnosed as stress or depression.

Dementia, like all serious long-term medical conditions, affects not just the people themselves, but their families and carers as well. Though people with dementia in all age groups face many of the same problems, younger people diagnosed with early-onset dementia have distinctive difficulties to face. They may still be working and have dependent children. They may have financial commitments, such as mortgages. They may be physically fit and have to deal with the social stigma and lack of understanding caused by their occasional unusual behaviour. In its early stages, early-onset dementia may cause quite subtle changes in behaviour that aren't immediately obvious to outsiders, so it may be hard for those with dementia and their carers to explain what's wrong. Plus, there's the psychological distress of realizing that, as one person put it, 'this disease is taking me away'.

Help is available for those with dementia and their families and carers, but provision is sometimes patchy, in spite of the government's new National Dementia Strategy, launched in February 2009. This promised £150 million over the first two years, with the aim being to:

- increase awareness of the problem;
- ensure early diagnosis; and
- improve the quality of care.

Much of the help, and many of the facilities provided are, understandably, aimed at older people and may not be appropriate for those diagnosed in their forties and fifties. However, there is specialized help out there, not only from statutory agencies but also from charities and campaigning groups like the Alzheimer's Society and those set up to support people with lesser-known dementias such as Pick's disease and Huntington's.

No-one would pretend that a diagnosis of early-onset dementia is anything but a blow – but there *is* still a life to be lived, for both those with dementia and carers. Making the most of it is what this book is about . . .

1

What is dementia?

Dementia – or, more properly, the dementias – is the name we use to describe a number of conditions which cause nerve cells to die in particular areas of the brain. As yet, researchers have been unable to find out exactly why this happens. However, the result is that the person affected gradually loses the ability to function effectively in the world. Memory loss is an early symptom of some dementias. This doesn't just mean the occasional absent-mindedness we're all familiar with – forgetting for a moment where we left our keys or glasses or the name of an acquaintance we meet on the street. It means the inability to remember who we are, our place in the world, how to perform the simplest of tasks like getting dressed or making a cup of tea, or how we should relate to those around us.

This is, of course, why dementia is so distressing for the families and loved ones of those affected. People with dementia will *look* familiar but may be unable to recognize their own family, may undergo personality changes, for example becoming rude or aggressive, and may behave in ways which would have horrified or embarrassed them in the past. Those with moderate to severe dementia will almost certainly need full-time care, whether this is provided in their own home or in a care home with special facilities for those with dementia.

Dementia is much more common in older people. It's now estimated that one in five of the over-85s has it to some degree, and that around one in three of us will die with it. As the population ages and medical advances mean that more and more of us live into our eighties, nineties and beyond, the issue of appropriate care for those with dementia will be spotlighted more and more.

Sadly, dementia is not *just* a problem for the very old and their families. Around one in 1,000 people under 65 will be affected by some form of the condition. People with early-onset dementia, as it's known, have particular difficulties to face. As we saw in the Introduction, they may have financial worries and dependent children. Both they and their families will also have to come to terms with the loss of the ability to remember, speak and understand the world around them at an age when they might have expected to lead a very different life. Dementia can be more aggressive in younger people, and is also more likely to be the result of some kind of genetic mutation, than dementia which develops in later life. Although the causes of dementia have not yet been fully identified, most researchers seem to feel that a combination of genetic and environmental factors leads to the development of the condition – or conditions, in the plural.

Dementia is very much an *individual* condition which affects different people in different ways. Some dementias seem to produce slightly different symptoms – for example, personality and behavioural changes rather than memory loss – depending on the area of the brain which becomes affected. Symptoms also tend to vary with time, especially in the early stages of disease, with people having 'good' and 'bad' days. This is, of course, difficult and frustrating both for those affected and for carers.

Alzheimer's disease is the most common form of dementia. In fact, the terms 'dementia' and 'Alzheimer's' are sometimes taken to be the same thing, although this isn't the case. About a third of those diagnosed with early-onset dementia have Alzheimer's. Some of those who develop Alzheimer's in middle age have the rare 'familial' form, which can be inherited. Children of affected parents have a 50 per cent chance of developing it too. However, the majority of cases of Alzheimer's are not of the type that can be inherited.

The condition causes the nerve cells in the brain – neurons – to degenerate, and disrupts the transmitters which carry messages in the brain. People with Alzheimer's produce less of the vital brain chemical acetylcholine. This is a neurotransmitter which carries messages and instructions between brain cells, enabling them to communicate. The regions of the brain which are especially affected by Alzheimer's include the temporal lobe and the hippocampus, which are the areas responsible for both the storage and the retrieval of new information. As these nerve cells are destroyed and die, the person gradually loses the ability to make decisions, to remember, to speak and to think logically.

An examination of the brain of someone with Alzheimer's disease after death will reveal that it has shrunk, that gaps have appeared in the affected areas, and that characteristic 'neurofibrillary tangles' and 'plaques' composed of fragments of an abnormal substance called beta-amyloid protein can be seen in the damaged parts of the brain.

As far as is known, there is no way to prevent the development of either early-onset or late-onset Alzheimer's. The characteristic changes that take place in the brain are not a normal part of ageing. However, a healthy lifestyle may help to reduce the risk, and anyone concerned about developing dementia will be advised to eat a healthy diet, low in saturated fats and rich in fruit and vegetables. In April 2010, American researchers reported the results of a four-year study of more than 2,000 older people and found that those who ate plenty of fish, poultry, fruit, nuts and dark leafy greens had a one-third lower risk of developing Alzheimer's than those who ate lots of meat, high-fat dairy products and butter. Make sure you are around the correct weight for your height, give up smoking and follow 'safe drinking' guidelines, and take regular exercise. Keeping your mind active, for example by reading, doing crosswords and having plenty of hobbies and interests, is also recommended.

Recent research has indicated there may also be a link between high blood pressure and dementia. A study at the University of Alabama looked at 20,000 people over the age of 45 and found that those with high diastolic blood pressure – the second figure in a blood pressure reading of, say, 140/90 – were more likely to have what is known as 'mild cognitive impairment'. This means they had problems with memory. Having regular checks and taking steps to reduce blood pressure if it's too high would seem to be a sensible precaution.

Vascular dementia, where damage to the blood vessels leads to the brain being deprived of oxygen, can also lead to the death of brain cells and cause dementia. There are actually two types of vascular dementia. One is stroke-related. It can involve damage to a particular part of the brain caused by a single stroke, in which case it is called single-infarct dementia. Dementia can also be caused by a series of mini-strokes, in which case it is known as multi-infarct dementia. Some areas of the brain are more affected than others, and as the strokes can be very slight and with few symptoms, the effects are variable. Deterioration may happen in small steps as one mini-stroke follows another. Depression, mood swings and sometimes epilepsy can result from vascular events.

The second type is caused by damage to the blood vessels deep inside the brain. Risk factors for this type of dementia are much the same as those for coronary artery disease and stroke illness. Smoking, high blood pressure, obesity, lack of exercise, high blood cholesterol levels and being diabetic can all predispose people to vascular disease.

There are also rarer forms of dementia which are especially likely to affect younger people, such as Pick's disease, sometimes known as fronto-temporal dementia, which usually strikes between the ages of 50 and 60, and Huntington's disease, a hereditary disorder of the central nervous system in which symptoms can develop at any time after the age of 30. Creutzfeldt-Jakob disease (CJD), a new variant of which hit the headlines in the 1990s after the BSE scandal, is caused by an infectious agent called a prion which attacks the brain and destroys the neurons. Other conditions such as HIV & AIDS, Parkinson's disease, multiple sclerosis and alcohol abuse can also lead to mild dementia or 'cognitive impairment' in their later stages, although this does not always happen. People born with learning disabilities such as Down's syndrome are especially likely to develop dementia in later life as well.

People with Pick's disease, like those with Alzheimer's, have deposits of abnormal proteins in their brains, although they are not the same proteins – those affecting people with Pick's are known as 'tau' and 'TDP 43'. Researchers have found that this form of dementia is 50 per cent triggered by an abnormal gene. Once it has been triggered, and it is not yet known how this happens, the brain is affected by the protein deposits. Neurons in different parts of the brain are then destroyed. People may lose their speech or be unable to remember the meanings of words. Pick's disease tends to lead to personality and behavioural changes and the inability to empathize with other people, rather than memory loss, as with Alzheimer's, but is equally distressing both for those affected and for their families.

Huntington's is a progressive neurodegenerative disorder caused by a faulty gene on Chromosome 4, which was discovered as recently as 1993. This leads to nerve cell damage in particular areas of the brain called the basal ganglia and cerebral cortex. The cells then die, causing physical, mental and emotional changes in the person affected. Huntington's can affect movement as well as thinking processes, leading to twitching, mumbling speech, clumsiness and – not surprisingly – stress and depression. Huntington's runs in families, with a 50–50 chance that the children of affected parents will inherit it. It is known that symptoms usually begin to show between the ages of 30 and 50.

The new variant of CJD mostly affected young adults who had eaten BSE-infected beef products. However, there are other types of CJD. 'Classical' CJD is much more common than the others and tends to affect the over-fifties. There is also an inherited form of the disease affecting younger people.

Some people have developed CJD after medical procedures such as treatment with human 'growth hormone' or, in very rare cases, a blood transfusion. Precautions have now been taken to minimize the risk of this happening: for example, all surgical instruments used on people with CJD are destroyed after use, and growth hormone is produced synthetically. CJD is not infectious in the way a cold or flu is, so there's no risk in normal social contact with those who have it. New variant CJD seems mostly – though not always – to affect young adults. Like other dementia-type illnesses, it leads to mood changes, memory loss, clumsiness, slurred speech and, later, to the loss of most ordinary functions. People with CJD tend to have a shorter life expectancy than those with other kinds of dementia.

Yet another form of dementia, known as 'dementia with Lewy bodies' or Lewy body dementia, is actually very rare in younger people. Like Alzheimer's, it is associated with protein deposits in nerve cells which damage them. As yet why this happens is not known. The so-called 'Lewy bodies' are also found in the brains of people with Parkinson's disease and the symptoms may be similar.

Dementia-type symptoms may also develop in people who have abused alcohol over many years. This can lead to memory loss, difficulty in learning and mood alterations and is often difficult to distinguish from the early stages of Alzheimer's disease. It's caused by a lack of thiamine – Vitamin B1 – which is essential to the production of the neurotransmitter acetylcholine. Unlike with dementia, however, it is sometimes possible to reverse the mental effects of heavy drinking if the person gives up alcohol and eats a healthy diet.

People with other conditions, such as HIV & AIDS, multiple sclerosis and Parkinson's disease, can also develop what is known as 'cognitive impairment' as a part of their illness, and find it difficult to remember things and to cope with everyday life. It's estimated that about one in five of those living with HIV develop some kind of cognitive impairment. This may lead to memory loss, lack of interest in the world around them, mood swings and difficulty in concentrating, though doctors now say that as more and more people with HIV are being treated with more effective drugs, these symptoms may become less common.

Parkinson's disease also involves damage to brain cells, but in a different part of the brain, the substantia nigra, which is involved in the organization of movement, leading to slowness, stiffness and shaking. Although having Parkinson's does increase your risk of developing dementia in later life, early-onset dementia is almost never associated with Parkinson's.

Multiple sclerosis is a progressive disease, and some people – around 45–65 per cent, according to the Multiple Sclerosis Society – do develop some type of 'cognitive difficulty' as it progresses. Memory lapses, problems with concentration and mood swings are not uncommon but they are not usually as severe as those experienced by people with Alzheimer's, for example. The term 'dementia' is not appropriate as most people experience only mild to moderate difficulties, sometimes finding it hard to read, follow conversations, plan and organize their lives.

Motor neurone disease is another progressive neuro-degenerative disease which causes weakness and wasting in the muscles, loss of mobility and problems with speech, swallowing and breathing. In most cases it doesn't cause cognitive difficulty but, according to the Motor Neurone Disease Association, about one in five people who have it are affected by some kind of personality change. This may be so slight it is almost unnotice-able, or it may lead to quite marked changes. A rare form of the disease – about 3 per cent of all cases – is associated with early-onset dementia.

It is also worth remembering that dementia-type symptoms can also be caused by treatable conditions such as thyroid prob-lems and vitamin deficiency.

People with learning difficulties, for example those born with Down's syndrome, are also more likely to develop dementia. The Alzheimer's Society says that about one-fifth of those with learning disabilities have Down's. About 2 per cent of people with Down's develop dementia in their thirties, rising to just over half (54 per cent) who develop the condition in their sixties. Researchers have discovered that almost everyone with Down's develops Alzheimer's-type 'plaques' in their brain, though not all of them develop dementia symptoms. As yet, we don't know why. The amyloid protein which, as we have seen, is found in these plaques is known to be linked to a gene on Chromosome 21. People with Down's have an extra copy of Chromosome 21, which explains the link. More research is clearly needed into why this happens.

People with other types of learning disability, and also those who have suffered a brain injury, are four times as likely to develop dementia as the general population.

Professor Martin Rossor of the Dementia Research Centre at the National Hospital for Neurology and Neurosurgery in London says that research into all the degenerative brain diseases overlaps, so that experts researching, for example, Alzheimer's, can often offer insights into other dementias too. As he says,

We can't look at a human brain and do a biopsy in the same way as we can on a liver or a stomach. But we can now look at the proteins which go wrong. They play a key role as they are the building blocks of cells. The shape of the proteins is important to their biological function. Degenerative diseases are often caused by these proteins becoming abnormally folded and the wrong shapes. Once this has happened it is hard for the brain to get rid of them or to grow new healthy ones.

We now know there are a whole host of proteins which are going wrong. Once one goes, others often do too, and diseases begin to overlap. We can learn from Alzheimer's, Parkinson's and motor neurone disease, as they progress. Some gene mutations we know can cause *either* Pick's or motor neurone disease.

At least seven different proteins have now been identified and research into motor neurone disease is helping us to understand why cells die. MRI scans can show us where brain cells are being lost. Different diseases only affect particular parts of the brain and different symptoms will appear, depending on where exactly in the brain the problem is.

Genetics and dementia

The part played by genes in the development of various kinds of dementia is complex and varied – and still not completely understood, though it is being extensively studied. For example, medical research has so far identified three genes which influence the development of early-onset Alzheimer's disease, known as the APP gene, PSEN-1 and PSEN-2. However, these genes are very rare, and account for fewer than one in 1,000 cases of Alzheimer's disease.

We all have between 50,000 and 100,000 genes contained on the 23 pairs of chromosomes which make up our individual genetic blueprint. Changes in genes which can cause disease are known as mutations. Our genes come in pairs and we inherit one copy from each of our parents. In some conditions, such as Huntington's disease, only one copy of the faulty gene is needed for the condition to be inherited. Others need two copies, one from each parent. Some conditions are influenced by more complex genetic factors; for example, mutations in several different genes can lead to the inherited form of Alzheimer's disease. However, most forms of dementia occur in people with no family link.

Genetic testing

If you have a strong family history of dementia, especially if it developed early in life, for instance between the ages of 30 and 60 in close family members, you might want to consider genetic testing. This will involve a laboratory analysis of your DNA from a blood sample, looking for the mutation or mutations which could lead to the development of dementia. Genetic testing can be used to:

- confirm a diagnosis;
- assess a person's risk of developing dementia, although having some of the faulty genes linked with Alzheimer's, as an example, cannot predict when or even if you will develop the condition;
- assess your risk of passing on a known inherited condition such as Huntington's disease to your children.

If you are considering genetic testing, you will need to ask your GP or consultant to refer you to a Regional Genetics Clinic. As well as offering you a test and help to make the decision whether or not to be tested, you should also be given specialist counselling and support.

There is a lot to think about before you decide that genetic testing would be of benefit, and in Britain you have to be over 18 to make the decision to be tested. The advantage of being tested for something like Huntington's is that it removes uncertainty and you can begin to make plans for the future. On the other hand, knowing that you will, at some unspecified point in the future, develop an untreatable and ultimately fatal disease is extremely distressing and hard to come to terms with.

There are implications for the rest of the family. Will they also want to know what is in store? There will be practical issues to consider and the possibility of discrimination in things like employment, mortgages, education, even life insurance. If the result is positive you will have conflicting emotions to deal with, ranging from guilt, shock and blame to anger and depression. Help from a specially trained genetic counsellor should enable you to learn more about the inherited conditions which can cause dementia and also to think carefully about the risks and benefits associated with being tested. Whether it is the right course for you will depend on your individual circumstances. If you do test, a counsellor can also help you cope with the results.

2

Getting a diagnosis

It was Laura who began to feel that there was something wrong. She was in her early fifties when she started 'losing' words and couldn't complete a conversation. She began to lose some other skills too – for example, she had trouble getting dressed and would often end up with her clothes on back to front or inside out. I took her to the GP, who thought at first that she might have an under-active thyroid. Eventually we saw a specialist at our local hospital and she was diagnosed with posterior cortical atrophy, the form of dementia author Terry Pratchett has.

Now she has trouble opening doors and using the telephone. She still reads the paper every day though she can't tell me what she has read. I have taken over household jobs like the cooking and the ironing. Laura is a happy soul who still loves going for long walks and shopping and holidays – we are planning a cruise this year. She is taking the drug Aricept but I know this will not cure her, only hold back the progress of the disease. We just live from day to day, that's all you can do.

Because early-onset dementia is a relatively rare condition, it's not always easy to obtain an accurate diagnosis. Indeed, many people find that a diagnosis is hard to obtain even when they are older and at increasing risk, partly because GPs are not always familiar with the signs and symptoms and partly because they feel that as there is no cure yet, nothing can be done to help.

However, this is far from being the case. With early-onset dementia in particular, it's important to obtain an accurate diagnosis as soon as is practically possible, because the drug treatments which exist – for example, for treating Alzheimer's disease – are only effective in slowing down the progress of the condition in its early stages.

- Any treatments offered need to take into account the type of dementia. For example, someone at risk of vascular

dementia will benefit from having symptoms such as atherosclerosis (the furring-up of the arteries with fatty deposits
which can lead to stroke illness) treated with blood-thinning
drugs.

- Anyone diagnosed will want to make plans for his or her
future care, including things like telling family, friends and
work colleagues and making arrangements for dealing with
personal affairs when he or she is no longer able to do so,
by setting up a Lasting Power of Attorney, for example. (For
more details of these practical steps, see Chapter 6.)

It's generally agreed that there need to be improvements in
early diagnosis – research in America suggests that even with
increasing openness about Alzheimer's and similar conditions,
obtaining a diagnosis can still take three or four years. Because
other dementias are less common, doctors see fewer cases and
are less likely to recognize the signs and symptoms. A single
visit, even to a specialist, may not be enough. Follow-up
appointments are important because those with degenerative
diseases get worse, unlike, for example, former stroke patients
whose condition may improve with time and treatment.

Most people associate dementia with memory loss and confusion, and it's true that this is one of the most common
symptoms. However, it's not the only one, and it is also worth
remembering that memory loss can also be associated with
other health problems, many of which are treatable. Being a bit
forgetful or confused does not automatically mean you have, or
will develop, dementia.

Symptoms to look out for

Many people with early-onset dementia and carers say that the
first sign they noticed that something was wrong was that the
person 'didn't seem quite him- (or her-) self'. In the early stages
of dementia, people may seem:

- to be forgetful or more absent-minded than usual;
- to tire easily;
- to find it hard to learn anything new;
- to behave in ways that seem strange or unlike them – for example, becoming more untidy or uncaring about their appearance when they have always been fastidious;
- disorientated in time and place, perhaps finding it difficult to remember a shopping list or even the way to the corner shop, or getting up for work when it's the weekend.

As the disease progresses it will become more and more obvious that this is more than just simple absent-mindedness. Memory lapses become more frequent and more serious. Short-term memory is often affected more than long-term. The person may be able to reminisce about his or her early years but totally forget what happened yesterday. Speech and language difficulties begin to be obvious, as the person forgets the names for common objects, loses his or her train of thought, does not complete sentences, or repeats what has already been said. He or she may ask the same question over and over, even when the answer has already been given several times.

'Motor' activities begin to be affected too, and the person has problems walking about, finding the way from bedroom to kitchen, putting on clothes in the right order. He or she has trouble recognizing objects and people (and of course this is always particularly distressing for carers and families). Slowly, he loses the ability to take care of himself or to make plans and organize his life. Someone living alone may neglect herself, leave the oven on or the front door open, get up in the night and wander off, 'forget' how to prepare or eat a meal or demand another because she doesn't remember she has already eaten, forget to pay bills or be unable to remember what the telephone is for, or how to use it.

Depression, aggression and frustration may be part of the illness as the person finds it hard to come to terms with what is happening. Dementia affects different people in different ways according to their original personality. Some became extremely cantankerous and difficult to live with; others are gentle and amenable. The tragic thing for families and carers is to see the person they once knew slowly disappearing and becoming an eccentric or aggressive stranger.

We shall be looking at the best way to manage these emotional and behavioural changes in detail in later chapters, but it's clear that long before this point is reached, it is vital to obtain a proper diagnosis so that a care plan can be worked out.

Who can help?

Your first port of call should be your GP, as soon as you begin to be sure that something is seriously wrong. Remember, once again, that many of the symptoms of early-onset dementia can be caused by other conditions. When your GP makes a diagnosis, one of the first aims is to eliminate all the other possibilities.

Because neither families nor GPs expect dementia to develop in younger people, the condition is often misdiagnosed as stress or depression, as it has some features in common. Someone who seems to undergo personality changes in mid-life, perhaps becoming more irritable, sad, anxious or agitated, may indeed be depressed – and may have reasons for being depressed. Physical illness, redundancy, children leaving home (the so-called 'empty-nest syndrome') or a general feeling that youth is gone and there's nothing to look forward to, can all contribute to the 'mid-life crisis' we hear so much about. Depression and anxiety can both be treated, either by very effective modern anti-depressant drugs or by 'talking therapies' such as cognitive behaviour therapy.

Confused behaviour can also be the result of other conditions, for example an under-active thyroid gland. Again, this can be treated, this time with hormone therapy. Vitamin deficiency, certain infections, the side effects of some drug treatments, extreme dehydration and in some cases brain tumours can all cause similar symptoms which can be mistaken for dementia. All these possibilities need to be investigated and eliminated before a definite diagnosis can be given.

Persuading the person that help is needed . . .

. . . is not always easy! We all know family members and friends who are reluctant to go to the doctor, no matter what their current state of health. Not surprisingly, when dementia is an issue great tact is necessary to persuade a loved one that a health check is really needed. The person may be perfectly aware that something is wrong, but be terrified of what the future holds if dementia is diagnosed. On the other hand, he or she may be in denial and insist that 'I am quite well' or 'I don't want to bother the doctor'. People can become quite skilled in covering up any memory lapses in the early stages of the condition, or are embarrassed at the mere suggestion that there is something amiss with their mental health.

Obviously you can't drag someone to the doctor if they refuse to go. If you're in that position, try phoning the GP's surgery and explaining what the problem is. Your GP might suggest dropping in informally to see you, or that you accompany your partner, friend or family member for a 'health check-up' for *both* of you. Alternatively, you could take advantage of any other health problem the person might have, such as flu or a stomach upset, to persuade him or her that a visit to the GP is necessary.

It took three years before Julia's husband was diagnosed with Pick's disease, aged 49. He had flatly refused to go to their GP.

I knew something was wrong when we were setting off to go to our daughter's graduation ceremony and he asked me where we were going. He had been behaving strangely for some time, commenting loudly on the appearance of strangers he saw on the bus, and barging past people without seeming to notice. He just wasn't the man I knew at all. In the end, I said that the doctor wanted to see us both, because I am diabetic, and this persuaded him to come along. After various tests he was referred to a psychiatrist and eventually diagnosed with Pick's, which I had never heard of. Since then we have had a lot of help from our community psychiatric nurse, who has been wonderful.

Sometimes the issue of 'patient confidentiality' is raised. Opinions vary on this and it's a decision only you can make, with the help of the medical professionals involved. Most people – whether on their own behalf or a loved one's – say that they *want* to know what is wrong, however gloomy the prognosis. But this isn't true for everyone. Many doctors like to talk to the person and carer or family member both together and separately, and this may be a good solution. Degenerative brain diseases affect everyone in the family, not just the person with the condition.

What your GP needs to know

Where dementia is suspected, input from family and friends is obviously extremely important in reaching a correct diagnosis. A GP consultation will be brief – at least initially – and the people who see the person every day will be far better placed to describe the symptoms and the deterioration or personality and behavioural changes they have noticed. It really helps if you write everything down before you get to the doctor's surgery so that you can give as accurate a picture as possible of the person's state of mind. Remind yourself when the symptoms started to appear and what was the first thing you noticed.

It can help, when you first suspect something might be wrong, to keep a 'symptom diary'. Is the person forgetful, irritable, depressed or anxious? Are these emotions and behaviours new to him or her? Is it possible that any medication, including anything recently prescribed, could account for the mood changes? Do the symptoms seem to be getting worse gradually, or do they vary day by day? All these details can be helpful when your GP is making a diagnosis or deciding whether to refer the person to a specialist for a second opinion.

How dementia is diagnosed

Dementia, as we have seen, can be caused by many different conditions, and dementia-type symptoms like confusion can occur in people who are actually suffering from something else entirely. As early-onset dementia is relatively rare, it may not even be suspected in a younger person. The Brain and Spine Foundation (contact details on p. 107) says that obtaining an accurate diagnosis is rather like doing a jigsaw. It's a matter of collecting the pieces and putting them together in the right order.

This means that many people who have early-onset dementia, and their carers, complain that getting a diagnosis has been a real struggle. Neurological symptoms are often hard to distinguish, and if your GP refers you to a specialist you may have to wait for an appointment and then wait for the necessary investigations. When in early 2009 the government announced that they wanted to see 'memory clinics' in every town and earmarked a generous £150 million towards setting them up, one government minister admitted that, at present, diagnosis could take as long as three years, which is clearly not satisfactory.

Patricia's husband was diagnosed with dementia in 2002.

Cyril had become very bad-tempered and was forgetting how to do very simple things, like open his attaché-case. Our GP told us he was depressed, but I had a feeling that wasn't the problem. We were shunted between old-age psychiatrists and neurologists, notes were lost between departments, and one specialist had Cyril in for tests lasting a whole day which were very tiring and distressing for him – in fact he ended up in tears. Eventually we did manage to see someone more sympathetic who allowed him to take breaks. It took about a year before dementia was diagnosed and by that time it was a relief to know exactly what was wrong.

Unfortunately there isn't, at present, a simple test which can tell you or your GP that this is definitely dementia. Usually the doctor will take a medical history and examine the person before applying a series of tests, most of which are devised to exclude other possibilities. For example, your GP will check for high blood pressure, ask whether the person is a smoker, and find out whether he or she has poor circulation, diabetes or high blood cholesterol levels. Any of these might indicate that atherosclerosis (furred-up arteries) could be putting the person at risk of a stroke or of vascular dementia. Tests for an under-active thyroid may also be carried out, as this condition can cause symptoms such as memory loss, confusion, depression and problems with concentration. Hypothyroidism, as it's known, can be treated with drugs.

A simple test called the MMSE – mini mental state examination – may also be applied to give some idea of the person's mental condition. This could involve asking the person:

- to say what the date is, or the name of the town or city;
- to repeat a simple sequence of words;
- to count back from 100 in sevens;
- to look at objects such as a pen or watch, and name them;
- to fold a piece of paper according to instructions, copy out a simple sentence or draw, for example, a clock face.

Depending on the results of these tests, the person may then be referred to a specialist. This may be a psychiatrist, ideally one with knowledge of early-onset dementias, or a neurologist. In 2007, it was said that 70 per cent of GPs were able to refer their patients to a 'memory clinic' for further investigations. Memory clinics are staffed by expert neurologists and nurses, who can offer neuro-psychological testing, drug treatments if appropriate, blood tests and also counselling, support and even carers' courses for families and friends.

Experts like neuro-psychologists have devised more sophisticated tests to aid diagnosis, as Dr Seb Crutch of the Dementia Research Centre explains.

Our job is to identify and corroborate the cognitive problems the person is having. We then ask whether he or she meets the established criteria for Alzheimer's or another type of dementia. We ask what the symptoms are and whether they are changing or getting worse, and then try to help patients and carers to understand what is happening.

We use tests of reasoning, diagrams, tests of the person's memory for events, facts, understanding and speech. Someone with Alzheimer's may struggle with visual problems, like not being able to see a hand in front of their face. Those with frontal lobe dementias may not be able to understand words but may still be very good at Sudoku. This is why outsiders sometimes think nothing is wrong – much of the person's ability remains.

Tests have also been devised to measure things like inhibition, decision-making and language. We build up a picture of the person by asking questions to test various different skills. For instance, if we show a picture of a dog, the person needs to be able to see the picture, to know what it is, to know its name, and to be able to say 'dog'.

All the time, we are also trying to take into account the person's previous ability, the severity of their illness, how hard the test is, whether they have any other impairment such as deafness, how old they are, what sort of mood they are in, and their level of fatigue or alertness. So diagnosis is a complicated process!

Further investigations could include a CT (or CAT), MRI or SPECT scan or an EEG, which are all ways of taking a more detailed look at what is happening in the brain.

A **CT (computerized axial tomography) scan** uses X-rays and computer technology to build up a series of pictures of cross-sections of the person's brain. It is usually done on an outpatient basis and may take anything from 15 to 30 minutes, during which the person has to lie quite still while the scanner takes a series of images. Results are not available immediately, but will be sent to your GP and/or specialist. They should show if the person has had a stroke, if there is a tumour on the brain, or if some of the changes characteristic of Alzheimer's disease can be seen. A CT scan is also useful in enabling the doctors to see whether the person may have another type of dementia.

An **MRI (magnetic resonance imaging) scan** is also a diagnostic tool but works in a slightly different way. Instead of using X-rays, like a CT scan, it uses magnetic resonance imaging, where a strong magnetic field and radio waves are used to produce images of the brain. MRI scans can show more detail than CT scans but they do take longer and, as with a CT scan, the person has to lie very still while the images are taken. The scanner can be noisy and some people find it claustrophobic. Not all hospitals are equipped with MRI scanners; they are expensive and require specially trained staff.

A **SPECT (single photon emission computerized tomography) scan** is a way of measuring blood flow through the brain. A very mild radioactive substance is injected into the bloodstream, and the person then has to sit still while the scanner takes pictures as this radioactive substance travels to the brain. The scan shows the doctor how well the blood is flowing in the brain and if there are any blockages.

An **EEG (electroencephalogram)** records the electrical activity of the brain, and is produced by attaching a number of electrodes to the person's scalp. Some of the rarer forms of dementia, for example Creutzfeldt-Jakob disease, produce characteristic brainwave patterns which can be identified by this particular test. A lumbar puncture, during which a sample of the cerebro-spinal fluid is drawn out from the lower back, can be used to help diagnose CJD by eliminating other causes of infection or inflammation.

Nancy, whose husband Geoff didn't obtain an accurate diagnosis for two years, comments:

Doctors – even consultants – must really listen to what families have to say, as well as talking to the person. Our GP was very good and referred us to a neurologist, but he hardly spoke to me. Geoff had been having problems at work and had undergone personality changes – giving away handfuls of money to homeless street people, getting lost when he was driving, being totally unable to concentrate on reading a book – things that only his partner would notice. However, the consultant we saw said it sounded like depression and referred Geoff to a psychiatrist. She prescribed an anti-depressant which had a terrible effect on him. He was becoming aggressive, inventing things that really hadn't happened and falling asleep at work, where the occupational health doctor signed him off sick and suggested we asked for a second opinion. Eventually we were able to see someone at the National Hospital for Neurology in London, where they really *listened* to me, as well as Geoff. After an MRI scan, he was diagnosed with fronto-temporal lobe dementia.

3

Treatments for dementia

At the moment, there is no cure for dementia. However, this doesn't mean that nothing can be done to make life easier for people with dementia or those who care for them. We shall be looking at ways of *managing* the condition in Chapter 4. In recent years, new drugs have been developed which can at least help to slow down the progress of the disease in some cases. There are new drugs in the pipeline, as well as research into other forms of treatment which might become available in the fairly near future. Some of the other symptoms of dementia, such as anxiety or aggression, can also be treated with already existing drugs.

Professor Martin Rossor of the Dementia Research Centre in London is sometimes asked when there will be a cure for dementing diseases.

> We can cure infections, and trauma, but with chronic diseases, for example diabetes, arthritis and eczema, we can manage or alleviate the symptoms. I hope that within ten years we will be able to manage dementing diseases also. Progress will probably be made on Alzheimer's first, since it affects more people, and the insights we get from that will help us with other dementias too. Most research is done by drug companies who are clearly going for the biggest markets.

As Alzheimer's is the most common form of dementia, it's understandable that much research into treatment is focused on it, and that the newest drugs are most suitable for those with Alzheimer's – though, as we shall see, they may be helpful to people with vascular and other dementias also. More research is needed on this.

We have already learned that people with Alzheimer's have a reduced amount of the brain chemical acetylcholine, which allows nerve cells in the brain to pass messages to each other. Between 1997 and 2000, three new drugs called acetylcholinesterase inhibitors have come on to the market. They don't cure confusion or memory loss, but because they work by reducing the breakdown of acetylcholine they have been found to be quite successful in stabilizing some of the symptoms of mild to moderate Alzheimer's for a limited amount of time.

The first drug of this type to be introduced was donepezil (brand name Aricept). Next came rivastigmine (brand name Exelon), and after that galantamine (brand name Reminyl), which was originally derived from snowdrop and narcissi bulbs! All are licensed for use in this country. Until October 2010, NICE, the National Institute for Health and Clinical Excellence, recommended that they should only be prescribed on the NHS for the treatment of *moderate* rather than mild dementia. These guidelines were updated in October 2010, and the Chief Executive said that NICE was now able to make a positive recommendation for their use in mild dementia. This decision was, of course, warmly welcomed by the Alzheimer's Society and patient groups.

All three drugs are intended to help with common symptoms such as forgetfulness and confusion. They can slow the rate at which a person deteriorates, but they will not stop the condition eventually getting worse. Aricept and Reminyl may help those with vascular dementia as well as Alzheimer's. Exelon may help those with Lewy body dementia (rare in younger people) or Parkinson's disease, but not vascular dementia. More research is needed into exactly who will benefit from these drugs, and whether they might also be used to treat more advanced dementia.

Cyril, who was diagnosed with Lewy body dementia in 2002

when he was in his fifties, has been taking Exelon ever since and has found it very helpful.

It has given me my life back. I feel much more in control, and although it is not a cure it is a lot better than nothing! I had to retire from my job and my chief hobby, which was wood-turning, but I have taken up photography, been on an art course, and still enjoy gardening. I recently saw the neurologist for a check-up and he said that there had only been a very slight deterioration in my condition.

Like all drugs, these three can have side effects. It appears that Exelon has more of these than the other two, with around one in three people having to stop taking it because of stomach upsets, fatigue, insomnia or dizziness. They also take some time to have an effect and doctors will usually prescribe a low dose initially, increasing it if the drug seems effective and well tolerated.

A fourth drug, memantine (brand name Ebixa) has now become available to treat moderate to severe dementia and has recently been recommended for NHS use by NICE. This drug works in a different way. Basically it changes the way brain cells communicate with each other, and also alters the amount of the mineral calcium which is present in them. It is thought that there may be a build-up of calcium in the brain cells of those with Alzheimer's. Memantine blocks the effects of another brain chemical called glutamate, which can damage nerve cells. Research in the USA has suggested that a combination of Aricept and Ebixa is more effective than Aricept alone, and more research is needed on this.

New drugs are always in the pipeline, including American research on a 'humanized monoclonal antibody' which is intended to bind to, and then clear, the beta-amyloid protein plaques in the brains of those with Alzheimer's. In theory, this could actually reverse the effects of Alzheimer's rather than just slowing the progress of the disease. A small trial was taking place in 2008, but so far results have been inconclusive.

The acetylcholinesterase inhibitors such as Aricept and Reminyl are basically aimed at making the remaining brain cells in those with Alzheimer's work more effectively. Researchers are also trying to develop what are known as 'disease modifying drugs' which will actually slow the decline of the brain cells. About 25 of these new kinds of drugs are currently being trialled.

Some of the more distressing symptoms of dementia can be treated with already existing drugs. For instance, the anti-epilepsy drug carbamazepine can be used to treat symptoms such as agitation and aggression. The benzodiazepine Ativan, a tranquillizer, is sometimes used to treat anxiety in people who also have dementia. More controversial is the use of a class of drugs called antipsychotics, which are sometimes used to calm down people with dementia or to deal with difficult behaviour such as aggression. Recent research from King's College London revealed that these drugs can have serious side effects, including an increased risk of stroke, as well as worsening some dementia symptoms when used long term. This led to a government report, published in November 2009, which pledged to reduce the use of these drugs by two-thirds.

'People can be cared for without this medication,' says Jan Flawn of PJ Care, an independent provider of specialist nursing care for people with degenerative neurological disorders. 'Our patients have been taken off medication and their difficult behaviour managed in other, more effective ways so that their quality of life is improved.'

An interesting piece of research from the USA was reported in early 2010 as suggesting that certain anti-blood-pressure drugs called angiotensin receptor blockers, or ARBs, could more than halve the risk of developing dementia. A team at Boston University had studied more than 800,000 people in the USA taking these drugs and had found they had up to a 50 per cent less risk of dementia. The drugs seem to play a key role in delaying the onset of symptoms.

Prevention, of course, is a key aspect of research, and the possibility of a vaccine, as well as new drug treatments, has been raised by experts at the Dementia Research Centre, based in the Hospital for Neurology and Neurosurgery in London.

'Immunotherapy is an important and exciting avenue for dementia research,' according to Professor Clive Ballard, Director of Research at the Alzheimer's Society.

The idea of using the immune system to 'clear away' the amyloid plaques found in the brains of people with Alzheimer's seemed promising after research in mice found that it was possible to do this. The mice were immunized; their immune systems created antibodies, and amyloid plaques were *not* deposited. Unfortunately, human trials had to be halted in 2002 because of serious side effects in some participants. Their immune systems seemed to over-react and they developed inflammation of the brain. However, scientists are still trying to find a way of reducing the damage done by this toxic protein *without* triggering an excessive immune response, and synthetic antibodies are being trialled.

The International Conference on Alzheimer's Disease in the summer of 2009 reported on a possible way of targeting a different faulty protein. Further immunotherapy trials are now in progress. It has also been discovered that Reminyl, one of the drugs already used to treat Alzheimer's, also seems to stop beta-amyloid proteins sticking together to form damaging plaques.

With the less common dementias, while drug and other treatments can sometimes help with associated symptoms such as depression or involuntary movements, there are as yet no drugs that will actually reverse or slow the progress of the disease. Speech therapy, for example, can be helpful in dealing with the speech problems experienced by people with Pick's disease or other fronto-temporal dementias.

Some of the symptoms of Huntington's disease can be eased by drugs such as tetrabenazine, which can control unwanted movement, or sleeping tablets for insomnia. There is research into the possibilities of an antibiotic called menocycline, and also into the use of co-enzyme Q10, an anti-oxidant vitamin-like substance, to treat both Huntington's and Parkinson's diseases. In the future, stem cell research may allow healthy brain cells to be grown and transplanted into the brains of people with Huntington's.

Existing drugs can be used to help ease the symptoms of conditions like multiple sclerosis and CJD. One drug, riluzole, is already approved for use in the NHS to treat motor neurone disease and has been found to increase survival rates somewhat. The MND Association (contact details on p. 109) is funding a trial of lithium carbonate, a drug currently used to treat mood-related disorders. Results are expected in the summer of 2011. The Association also has details of other clinical trials currently taking place in Europe and the USA.

It's good news that money is at last being spent on research into these devastating diseases, as governments across the world realize that with an ageing population, all forms of dementia are going to become more prevalent. However, the Alzheimer's Research Trust (contact details on p. 107) points out that while £590 million is spent on cancer research every year, only £50 million goes to dementia research. In fact, for every £1 spent on dementia research, the country spends £26 on researching cancer and £15 on researching heart disease.

The Trust is currently supporting many research projects around the country. The work it has funded has already contributed towards a better understanding of the causes of Alzheimer's, including the discovery of two new Alzheimer's-related genes and more information about the amyloid protein which builds up in the brains of affected people.

Research is also being undertaken into attempts to improve

early diagnosis, with new tests already in the pipeline, including one which examines nerve cells at the back of the eye to see if any disease-producing changes can be seen. Work is also taking place on both prevention and treatment.

Professor John Hardy, a scientist running a laboratory which investigates neurodegenerative diseases, says:

> We are studying genetics because this leads us to better understanding of these diseases and because counselling can be offered to patients when genes are discovered. Research is more collaborative than it used to be and international data is being pooled so I am cautiously optimistic. We already know of two genes linked to the familial form of Pick's disease and one major gene on Chromosome 9 has still to be found.
>
> The more of the picture you have, the easier the research becomes as we are able to build up a picture of what a particular gene does, what its role in the brain is, and what is going wrong with it. It's rather like doing a jigsaw.
>
> Research has been helped by the human genome project. We can now do about five years' work in six months because we know the sequence of every gene. Stem cell biology is also useful. We are much better at making cells do new and different things. Dolly the sheep was developed from a skin cell, and the Alzheimer's Research Trust scientists are working on turning skin cells into nerve cells. So there are grounds for cautious optimism.

Non-drug therapies

Non-drug therapies can sometimes be useful in the early stages of dementia, but the results of trials seem so far to be inconclusive. Ginkgo biloba, a herbal remedy often used in traditional Chinese medicine, is said to improve brain and memory function, but there have been few reliable studies which prove its effectiveness. See Chapter 8 for more information about alternative and complementary treatments for dementia.

Speech and occupational therapy can, of course, be useful in dealing with some of the problems associated with some forms of dementia. As well as helping with speech and language itself, speech therapists can offer advice on the difficulties with feeding and swallowing which may be experienced as dementia progresses. Many occupational therapists specialize in working with people with dementia and can give both those with dementia and their carers useful tips on organizing their lives as memory begins to fail – things like keeping familiar objects in their usual places, labelling rooms and cupboards, and putting up photographs of friends and family, all clearly labelled with their names. (More about memory aids in Chapter 4.)

Exercise can help to lift mood, especially if the person has previously been keen on walking or sport. Multi-sensory stimulation, including lighting, sounds (including music), massage and aromatherapy, can be soothing. Some support groups for those with dementia include group discussions and 'reminiscence therapy', and also behaviour modification techniques as a way of coping with difficult or inappropriate behaviour. (More about support groups for those with early-onset dementia in Chapter 5.)

4

Dementia day to day

My husband was 49 when he was diagnosed with fronto-temporal dementia and he still doesn't know he is ill. His behaviour was beginning to alienate our grown-up children even before his diagnosis. He became totally self-centred, wouldn't listen to anything they said, and took no interest in his grandchildren. The children do support me but they won't come to the house because they can't cope with their dad.

He has since had a series of 'transient ischaemic attacks', like mini-strokes, and is a little less capable after each one. He sleeps for about four hours at a time and has no sense of night or day, so he complains if he isn't given a meal even if it's 3 a.m. He is on medication to reduce his agitation, but it's obvious to me that he is not happy and has no quality of life. He just sits and looks, or paces the floor, or asks repeatedly when he is going 'home' even though we have lived for 20 years in the same house.

We have a fantastic early-onset dementia co-ordinator here in Cambridgeshire who has set up support groups and arranged help for us. We have two regular and one occasional helper coming in. Alan needs to see the same people but I'm not sure he recognizes them. He doesn't recognize me. I've thought about respite care but I think he would be difficult to manage in unfamiliar surroundings, and probably worse when he came home again.

Gillian's story, above, illustrates just how difficult it can be to live with someone with early-onset dementia. Dementia is as individual as the people who have it. Not only do the symptoms of different dementias vary, as we have seen in earlier chapters, but so do the effects on individual personalities. Day-to-day management is different for everyone too. Some people may be suffering from no more than slight memory loss, get very tired or be unable to do all the things they once enjoyed. Others may become aggressive, frustrated, frightened or generally 'difficult'. It can be hard for husbands, wives and families, suddenly

31

transformed into 'carers', to remember that it's the *condition* that is the real problem, that the person you loved is still there underneath – however much changed – and that he or she may be more frightened, bewildered and unhappy than you are. Your loved one isn't forgetting the simplest instructions, shouting at you or wandering off just to make your life harder!

We shall be looking at the help available for families and carers in Chapter 7. It's also important to remember that dementia is a progressive condition and that in its later stages residential care may be the best and safest option for everyone. We shall be looking at residential care for those with early-onset dementia in Chapter 9.

While you are still living with someone with any form of early-onset dementia, you will need to learn how to manage the condition, and the difficult and sometimes distressing behavioural changes that go with it. This is where support groups, both nationwide organizations like the Alzheimer's Society (contact details on p. 107) and local groups for those with dementia and their carers, fulfil an invaluable role. Whatever your problem is, you can be sure that someone, somewhere, will have faced it before you and found a way to deal with it. You can too. The Alzheimer's Society website has an online forum where you can post details of the particular problem you are facing, and obtain responses from other people who have coped with the same thing.

Families find their own ways of dealing with the diagnosis and the difficulties that can arise in the early stages while everyone tries to come to terms with what has happened.

> My way of dealing with it is to laugh at it, even though I know it will take me away in the end.

> I tried to fight it, telling myself there had to be some mistake, but then it became more obvious.

> He gets very angry and frustrated when other people just don't see it. Friends keep saying that he's fine, which is hard because we know he isn't.

He has changed so much. He has become so introverted and doesn't speak much, because he is frightened of making a mistake. The sociable man I used to know seems to have lost interest in life.

The Alzheimer's Society's TV and press campaign, 'I have Alzheimer's . . . but I also have a life', fulfilled an important role by reminding the rest of us that those with dementia deserve to be treated with love and respect, whatever their symptoms. It's up to carers as well as the medical profession to help people with dementia retain their dignity, confidence, self-esteem and independence for as long as possible.

Memory loss

This is the symptom most commonly associated with the dementias, although not everyone with early-onset dementia has memory problems. Those who do may find that their symptoms vary quite a lot. Some are able to hang on to learned skills until the illness is quite advanced; others are not. Many people in the early stages of dementia forget what happened in the recent past but retain quite accurate memories from long ago. Creating a 'memory box' or scrapbook might be a good way to connect with someone who enjoys reminiscing.

Of course, it can be frustrating for carers to have to continually remind a loved one about simple, everyday tasks like taking a bath or finding the way to the shops. Experts recommend memory aids such as Post-it notes wherever they are needed. Health professionals such as occupational therapists can give carers advice on different memory aids, and simple everyday things like calendars and pinboards in prominent places can help people to remember what they are supposed to be doing at a particular time. Keeping to a regular routine can be reassuring. Make sure the same things are always in the same place in your home – house keys on the hall table, coffee mugs next to the kettle, pyjamas under the pillow. A change of location or even rearranging the furniture can be very confusing for someone who is losing his or her memory.

Don't pressurize the person by continually asking her if she can remember this or that; she is likely to become upset or flustered. Try to empathize with her feelings, rather than telling her she is wrong.

Some people can remember the distant past much more clearly than the immediate past. 'Reminiscence therapy' – looking at old photographs, playing familiar music and talking about the old days – may be helpful in the early stages of dementia. Others have problems taking in new information. The key to dealing with that is to keep the new information simple and repeat it as often as necessary; 'It's Tuesday, you always go to the Day Centre on Tuesday,' for example.

Forgetting names and faces is common and can, of course, be terribly distressing for friends and family. Carers can help by giving information like 'Here's Sue from next door to see you!' As the disease progresses and people become more and more confused, they may accuse their nearest and dearest of anything from stealing money or possessions to sexual molestation. Of course this is extremely upsetting but you have to remember it's the illness, not the person, which is responsible. You can help by giving reminders, when the person is more calm and relaxed, of who you are – and, indeed, who he or she is. Labels can be put on doors and cupboards to help with finding things in the house.

The Alzheimer's Society recommends breaking down necessary tasks like getting dressed or making a cup of tea into small, manageable steps. Carers should try and do things *with* the person, rather than *for* them. You'll need to retain a sense of proportion as well as a sense of humour. As one carer said, does it really matter if he insists on wearing his clothes to bed or prefers to eat with a spoon rather than a knife and fork? Better to let him have his way than for both of you to become distressed by continual arguments. If the person can only do part of the task him or herself, that's better than nothing. Even as the disease progresses, there will probably still be some simple household tasks he or she can help with – loading the washing machine, for instance, or sweeping up leaves in the garden.

People with memory loss need to be guided, not shouted at. Tact and encouragement are important too, as is maintaining, for as long as possible, hobbies and interests that they have always had. Exercise can help; going for a walk or even going to the gym or a gentle game of tennis or bowls can be cheering and soothing and prevent frustration.

Too much hustle and bustle, on the other hand, can be distracting. Give the person one thing at a time to concentrate on and try to keep to a recognizable routine so that he or she feels reassured and is able to enjoy life as much as possible.

'In the early stages of dementia it is important to keep hobbies and interests going if you can,' says one experienced occupational therapist. 'Obviously, it depends on the individual – some artists and musicians, for instance, feel they would rather give up than paint or play less well than they once could. However, that need not mean that they can no longer get pleasure from art or music.'

Because early-onset dementia is relatively rare, there may not be a lot of suitable facilities in your local area, but you may still be able to engage with the local community in some way. If your partner is a golfer, for instance, a chat to the committee of the local golf club might mean he or she could carry on and the other members make allowances. There's no reason why people with dementia should suddenly stop doing things they enjoyed. They may say they can't be bothered or begin to avoid social situations because of embarrassment, but if you are open and honest, friends and neighbours can be understanding. They need to be given a chance. If the local newsagent knows which paper your partner usually buys and where you live, she'll be able to send him home if he becomes lost or confused – and having to go and fetch the paper gives the person with dementia something to do.

It's tempting for the carer to 'take over' as it's often quicker and easier, but better for the person with dementia if he or she *can* keep busy, stay involved and take part in the decision-making process as far as possible.

Difficult behaviour

Dealing with 'difficult' behaviour – which can cover anything from out-and-out aggression to being asked the same questions over and over or inappropriate sexual touching – is one of the hardest parts of caring for someone with any kind of dementia. The ordinary, social rules of everyday life just don't apply. When you know that, before this illness, your loved one would have been horrified and humiliated by what he or she is doing, it can be both sad and stressful.

The keys to managing most kinds of difficult behaviour include *reassurance* and *distraction*. People with dementia can be very frightened and anxious, unable to understand what is happening to them or around them, and this can lead them to behave in unacceptable ways. Remember, it's the illness that is responsible, not the person. Whatever they are doing, they may be trying to communicate feelings and emotions that are very real to them. If you, as carer, can work out what these are, you may be able to help.

Aggression, for instance, can mean anything from threats and verbal abuse to minor or even quite major violence, or obvious agitation. The first thing to say is that if the person is seriously violent, you must get help – don't try to cope on your own.

Prevention is better than cure. If you can learn to recognize what it is that is causing the upset or anger, it may be possible to avoid the situation completely. Ask yourself if you absolutely *have* to do whatever it is – and whether you have to do it right now. If the person seems agitated and restless, he or she may be in pain, or may just need the loo, so this is something you should check out. If there is a violent episode, try to stay calm yourself or you might make matters worse. Take a deep breath, count to ten, even get out of the room if you have to. Don't argue and don't touch or try to restrain the person until he or she has calmed down, when a reassuring hug might be appropriate.

Once things are calmer, your loved one might very well forget the incident has ever happened, or alternatively pick up on your feelings of distress and seem anxious or upset him or herself. This is where reassurance comes in. Someone with dementia may need to be told, over and over, that everything is all right, that you are taking care of things, that all is well. Someone who is frequently aggressive or agitated might benefit from a short course of medication. Ask the advice of your GP, community psychiatric nurse (CPN) or specialist if this seems appropriate.

Try to imagine how confusing life must be for people with dementia. They may be aggressive because they don't understand what is happening or why they now need help with 'private' activities like washing or getting dressed or going to the lavatory. They may be anxious because there seems to be too much going on, or because they have no clear idea of where they are, who you are or what is expected of them, especially if you seem brisk or impersonal or critical. They may be in pain, need the loo or be hungry or thirsty. It can help to try and work out just what it is they are trying to communicate.

You can help by:

- sticking to a calm, stress-free routine as far as possible;
- explaining carefully what is required of them, and giving them time to take in what you say;
- guiding and helping rather than taking over – even though it may be frustrating for you!

- trying to focus on the things they can still do;
- being as patient as possible;
- learning to interpret their behaviour so that you can spot 'danger' signals and be ready to reassure;
- encouraging them to take exercise so that they are healthily tired at the end of the day, rather than bored and frustrated with pent-up energy.

Not everyone with dementia becomes aggressive, of course. Other kinds of behaviour that can be difficult for carers to cope with include repeating the same questions over and over, following you around, shouting and screaming, waking in the night, wandering off, hiding or losing their belongings, becoming suspicious and accusing you or other people of stealing from them or attacking them, and also inappropriate sexual behaviour. Again, it's worth remembering that other carers will have found ways of dealing with all this, and a 'visit' to an online forum such as the Alzheimer's Society's can offer a lot of insight. You can also share your concerns with your community psychiatric nurse or other people in a local carers' group.

Again, it can help if you manage to work out just *why* this particular kind of incident is happening. Repetitive behaviour, for example – pacing the floor or repeating the same movements and activities – can sometimes be the result of boredom. You could try giving the person something to do. Your loved one may be well enough to help you with a simple household task such as bed-making. One carer found her partner enjoyed doing children's jigsaw puzzles; another gave his wife a cardboard box to 'pack' and 'unpack' with small household items. Folding laundry or newspapers or 'painting' the garden fence with a bucket of water are also suggestions.

It can be particularly poignant if the person continually asks to go 'home' or demands to see a parent or relative who is no longer around. Here again, reassurance is the key. Tell her she is safe and cared for and, if necessary, you could walk her round the block and home again. Try to talk to her about 'Mum' or the brother she is asking for, instead of repeating the brutal truth that Mum actually died 30 years ago, which will only upset her further. Reassurance is also needed if she seems very insecure and keeps following you around. 'It's all right, love, I'm here, I'm not going anywhere, everything's fine,' is something you will almost certainly have to repeat, over and over again.

Many people with dementia find it difficult to differentiate between night and day and may get up in the small hours and try to leave the house. Make sure outer doors are locked, and if this happens lead your loved one gently back to bed, pointing out the time on the bedside clock. Check that he or she doesn't need the loo before going back to bed. Again, regular exercise through the day will encourage better sleep at night and make people less inclined to wander.

Shouting and screaming can be very upsetting for you, for the person you're caring for, and for the neighbours! Some people with dementia do have hallucinations and you will want to check with your GP or CPN to see if that is what is frightening your loved one. Sleeping with a night-light can help if darkness is upsetting. Removing a mirror from the room, so avoiding coming face to face with an unexpected 'stranger', can also help.

Hiding and losing things – a purse, keys, glasses – can make someone with dementia very agitated, and of course it's frustrating for carers too. Make sure you have spare copies of as many vital possessions as possible and keep spare keys and spare glasses in the same place all the time. It might be useful to have at least one cupboard with a lock so that vital papers and so on can be kept safe, especially if the person has a habit of throwing things into the dustbin or flushing them down the lavatory! As a carer you may have to get used to finding your loved one's possessions in unusual places – glasses hidden under sofa cushions, a saucepan in the bathroom – but you may also find that he or she has favourite hideaways which should be regularly checked out. Some people hoard food after getting confused about whether they have eaten or not, so it's important to be sure that anything perishable hasn't been secreted somewhere. Leaving something simple like a small packet of biscuits in a favourite hideaway might be enough to reassure the person that food is always available.

If your loved one accuses you – or anyone else – of stealing, or of molesting him or her, don't take it personally. Be reassuring, and provide distraction by offering something interesting to do, or a favourite TV programme to watch or a piece of music to listen to. (Of course, if you have any doubts about another carer or family member, do check them out. Sadly, abuse of the mentally infirm does sometimes happen.)

Distraction is also the best way to deal with overt and inappropriate sexual behaviour on the part of your loved one. Some forms of dementia do lead to what is known as 'disinhibition' which can cover things like undressing in public, exposing oneself, masturbation, or trying to touch or fondle complete strangers. Stay calm, give the person something else to do or think about, and explain to the 'victim', if there is one, that the person acting so inappropriately has dementia and doesn't mean to offend. The same applies if your loved one behaves in an anti-social way. Some forms of dementia seem to remove normal social constraints so that embarrassing incidents occur.

As one carer says,

> David behaves like a child. He just seems to say the first thing that comes into his head, like 'You're fat, aren't you? Why are you so fat?' to a lady in the doctor's waiting-room. Or when we go to the supermarket he just whizzes round with the trolley, bumping into people and displays, and barges into the queue at the checkout rather than waiting in line like everyone else.
>
> I explain to people that he can't help it, it's part of his illness, but as he looks perfectly all right I'm not sure whether they believe me. It's

easier to go to the shops when they're less crowded and there's less chance of a confrontation.

Safety

While it's important to allow people with dementia to retain as much independence as they can handle, it is also obviously important to make sure they are safe. Keeping the balance between the two is not always easy. You'll need to make sure that common-sense safety precautions are in place all round your home. Good lighting, smoke alarms, non-slip rugs, hand-rails on the stairs and grab-rails in the bathroom, night-lights if the person becomes agitated or wanders at night, locks on doors and cupboards, can all help to reduce the risk of accidents.

It's as well to keep a first-aid kit handy and be aware of what to do in case of minor injuries like burns, scalds, cuts and bruises. An occupational therapist will also be able to give you tips and hints on keeping your loved one safe at home. MedicAlert bracelets with all the necessary information about the person's condition can be obtained from <www.medicalert. org.uk>. It also makes sense to let neighbours, local shopkeepers and the police know if the person is inclined to wander, or go for walks and forget where he or she is.

Eating and drinking

A healthy, balanced diet containing foods from all food groups, low in saturated fats and sugar and including plenty of fruit and vegetables, is just as important for someone with dementia as it is for everyone else. As a carer, you will need to be calm and flexible and willing to help your loved one to enjoy food, whether or not this means feeding him or her. Some people with dementia lose interest in food or refuse to eat, which can be worrying. There may be a physical reason for this – they may have bad teeth or a painful mouth or difficulty in swallowing.

If this seems to be the case, you could ask to be referred to a speech and language therapist. It isn't as well known as it should be that these particular health professionals specialize in the care of the mouth and throat and will be able to suggest ways of encouraging a reluctant eater to eat again.

Depression can make people with dementia lose interest in food. If they don't get enough exercise they may not be very hungry. They may have forgotten how to chew or swallow or be unable to recognize the fact they are hungry. Alternatively, they may over-eat, perhaps because they have forgotten that they have already had a meal. This of course brings with it the risk of choking, or perhaps of putting on an unhealthy amount of weight.

The Alzheimer's Society can offer tips on helping people to eat well.

Incontinence

Not everyone with early-onset dementia is, or will become, incontinent, and certainly not in the early stages of their illness. If toileting does become a problem, you can ask your GP to be referred to a continence adviser, who will let you know how the condition is best managed.

Initially it may be enough to remind your loved one that he or she needs to go to the loo, and make sure this happens regularly. Carers often learn to recognize the signs – some people become restless, or fiddle with their clothing, when they need to be taken to the bathroom. A photo of the bath or the loo on the appropriate door can help them to orientate themselves.

Accidents do happen and can be humiliating and upsetting for both the person with dementia and the carer. Sometimes incontinence can be caused by medical conditions which can be treated, so a visit to the GP should be your first step. Urinary tract infections can be treated with antibiotics. Men in middle age can develop prostate problems which can also be treated. Some medication can cause side effects including incontinence.

Some people with dementia become very distressed when they have an accident and may hide their wet or soiled clothes. Others seem unaware there is a problem. For anything more than the occasional accident, incontinence aids like pads, pants and waterproof bedding are available. You can obtain details of these from your local continence adviser or the Bladder and Bowel Foundation (contact details on p. 107). Clothes that are easy to put on or remove – for example, trousers with elasticated waists rather than zips or buttons – may be easier for a confused person to deal with. Specially adapted clothing is available by mail order or from websites such as <www.allaboutinconti nence.co.uk>. If you, as a carer, find incontinence difficult or embarrassing to cope with, the continence adviser can help.

Hygiene is especially important when someone has incontinence as skin can easily become sore and uncomfortable. Skin should be washed with warm water and unscented soap or specialist skin washes, and then patted rather than rubbed dry. Finally, barrier cream should be applied. The Bladder and Bowel Foundation can advise on suitable hygiene and skincare products, many of which are available from supermarkets and high street pharmacies such as Boots.

5

Help for early-onset dementia

Although the major campaigning organizations like the Alzheimer's Society provide help and support for everyone affected by dementia whatever their age, they acknowledge that more specialist facilities are needed for those who have early-onset dementia. Their website mentions 'significant' age-related barriers for younger people trying to access dementia services. Much of the help provided is aimed at the over-65s who are, of course, the vast majority of people with dementia. Younger people tend to get 'lost'. This can mean that some, even if they are able to find support and day-care places, have needs that are not being met. Those in their forties or fifties when diagnosed have different needs, preoccupations and interests compared to those in their seventies or eighties.

Those with early-onset dementia will probably, for instance,

- still be working. How do they find out about their employment rights or about benefits if they become too ill to work?
- be physically fit and healthy;
- have younger families who need to be cared for and kept in the picture;
- have financial commitments such as a mortgage.

Those specializing in the care of older people with dementia may not be able to offer the right levels of expertise in dealing with these age-specific issues. So where do younger people and their carers find help?

Specialist NHS services

With increased attention being given to the rising numbers of people affected by dementia, there is more and better provision of specialist services than there has ever been. In 2006, it was estimated that there were 145 specialist services for younger people affected by dementia around the country. Back in 1996, there were only 20, so your chances of finding appropriate provision close to where you live have improved. However, the services are not evenly spread across the country and the amount of help they can provide will vary.

As an example, the Leeds Younger People with Dementia Team has been in existence since 1995 and works alongside a local branch of the Alzheimer's Society which runs a day centre and provides carer support.

Team member Dr Dearden explains:

> We see people for assessment and they are referred to us by GPs, Social Services and others. We have just over a hundred people on our caseload and manage their care from diagnosis right through to end-of-life. I know facilities vary around the country. Here in Leeds it's difficult to find appropriate respite or continuing care for younger people, who don't necessarily want to be cared for alongside much older people. The day centre, run by the local Alzheimer's support group, provides day care for younger people among their peers. Some of the people are still working so have work-related issues; some have young children, and there is an outreach team too.

As Dr Dearden says, the local branch of the Alzheimer's Society runs a day centre for younger people with dementia. The manager, Peter Ruickbie, says:

> It is partly therapeutic and partly social. We have to be proactive about the services we provide. We have two minibuses so we can offer trips out. There's a walking club, a gardening club, plus indoor activities such as films, a computer club, aromatherapy and hairdressing. The members decide on the activities they want – someone did a sponsored cycle ride from Land's End to

John O'Groats for us so they then had to decide how to spend the money raised.

Most of our members are in their fifties but we do have some younger people, especially as alcohol-related dementias seem to be on the rise. The dementias affecting younger people tend to lead to symptoms such as mood and personality changes rather than just memory loss. In addition, younger people with dementia have different lives from older people. Some have young families. The support we provide can allow partners and carers to work and pay the mortgage. We support carers and children so that they can carry on with their lives and also offer practical advice on things like benefits and Power of Attorney.

About a third of local people with early-onset dementia live alone and our community outreach project is another important part of our work. Our work with them is largely preventative, helping them to cope with staying in their own homes so they don't need to call on the emergency services. Support could mean anything from shopping and travel to helping people to take their medication.

People are usually referred to us from local memory clinic services – the part of the NHS dealing with mental health.

Local groups

Chris Wyatt is the area manager for the Alzheimer's Society in the South East. She describes local facilities for people with early-onset dementia as

very much user-led – the people involved let us know what they need! There is one particular group based in Woking called Gimmmicks which is a peer support group. They organize activities, go out, support each other, and are very vocal and aware.

They decide on the activities they want, which can be anything from a pub meal to a visit to a local place of interest. They organize events and other group activities and get great support from each other if any of the group are feeling down. Carers are often not involved except to the extent of bringing them along to the group. Originally they just met for two hours once a month, but now it's one day a week. They may just meet for coffee and read the newspapers or they may go out; usually between ten and 15 people attend.

Some of the group have Parkinson's-related dementia, other have Pick's disease or Lewy body dementia. The group is run very much by people with dementia for people with dementia, and they get the support they wish for. There is a link person who is a dementia support worker with knowledge and understanding of the various conditions but, as I've said, the service is very much user-led. Gimmicks started five or six years ago.

As far as we know there are about 1,500 people in the Surrey area with early-onset dementia. They are becoming increasingly vocal and want to feel ordinary and part of the community. Most don't mind other people knowing about their dementia.

We have another group who meet in pubs with their carers, and another which is a sort of supper club for those with dementia, carers and their wider families. Social activities are very important but local groups can also help with practical things like work and benefits, as well as issues around relationships.

It can be hard for partners to cope with early-onset dementia because it tends to strike at an age when couples are thinking about moving into a new phase of life – the children are becoming more independent and suddenly all their plans for the future have to change. Younger dementias tend to progress more quickly, which is another factor to take into account.

Groups do help people to find coping mechanisms because there is usually someone who has faced the same thing, who has perhaps had to leave work early, and found that their network of friends and family has completely changed. There is still some stigma attached to mental illness, but it's not just that. Friends may simply not know what to do or say or how to support someone with one of these conditions. Peer support for those with dementia and carers' support is often the basis for real friendships.

As well as emotional support from other group members, we run information sessions two or three times a year discussing all the issues – everything from incontinence, difficult behaviour, the law and Lasting Powers of Attorney to employment rights, separation and divorce – anything people might need to know. Support groups are an invaluable resource but there will never be enough of them – people will often have to travel further than is ideal! But we are there.

Community psychiatric nurses

Obtaining an accurate diagnosis can, as we have already seen, take time. Doctors, from GPs to specialists, will want to exclude the possibility of symptoms being caused by other conditions before they can definitely say that early-onset dementia is the problem. Once diagnosed you may be referred to a community psychiatric nurse.

Ian Hulatt is the mental-health adviser to the Royal College of Nursing. As he says,

> The CPN's job is to support the person with dementia and their carer. Every presentation of dementia is different and care plans have to be tailored to the person's individual needs – there is no 'off-the-shelf' plan. Sadly, increasing numbers of younger people are presenting with dementia because of hugely increased alcohol consumption, in addition to the other forms of dementia which affect younger people as well as the over-65s.
>
> A CPN will come to your home and assess your needs, looking at the person's ability to cope with the 'activities of daily living' – things like self-care, shopping and handling finances. People in the early stages can often manage very well with reminders such as diaries and Post-it notes. As the illness progresses, the CPN can often advise on things like food and eating, incontinence, mobility or any other problems which may arise. We can also advise on medication if it's needed, activity and comfort. Then in the later stages we can give information on night-sitters, respite care and eventually full-time care. The CPN will go on the journey with the person with dementia and his or her carer and support them right to the end of the person's life – and beyond, if the carer needs it.
>
> When it comes to challenging behaviour we may be able to help to explain why it is happening and what can be expected to happen, as well as offering strategies to help manage the behaviour. If necessary we can discuss whether medication might be appropriate so that both the person with dementia and the carer can get some sleep.
>
> A CPN will suggest distraction and diversion from stressful issues and help in handling problems, for example if the person

asks for 'Mum' when Mum has passed away many years ago. We know that repeated questioning can make carers irritable and frustrated – and sometimes guilty for feeling that way – and it's important that they acknowledge their feelings. A CPN is there for the carers too.

Occupational therapists (OTs) help people with dementia to keep their lives as normal as possible by offering assistance where it's needed with the activities of everyday living.

Heather is an OT specializing in the care of people with dementia. She feels that the guidelines in the latest government Dementia Strategy should enable OTs to be more proactive and intervene in personal care earlier, before problems actually start. As she admits,

> At the moment there's a tendency not to bring in the professionals until there is a problem. All NHS trusts work in a slightly different way so people with early-onset dementia may be diagnosed through a memory clinic, or may see a psychiatrist, a psychologist, a neurologist or all of them. Sometimes people are referred to us by the community mental-health team or by their GP. I would always recommend asking to be referred to an OT who is a specialist in dementia care.
>
> I always take a detailed case history and ask people what they are having difficulties with. It could be that they are not able to keep up with their workload. They may be losing their keys, forgetting names or unable to keep up on the golf course. Anxiety about their symptoms may play a part and can make their problems worse. I try to help them to stay calm and focused and recommend that they talk to their friends openly and honestly. Keeping the condition a secret can put great pressure on individuals, their family and friends.
>
> Care for people with dementia should become more person-centred. This means that instead of testing them to discover what they can no longer do, we work on their strengths and the things they *can* still do – and enjoy! I try to look at the person's everyday functioning and adjust when help is needed.

Memory clinics

In 2007, it was estimated that about seven out of ten English GPs were able to refer people with dementia to a local memory clinic. Two years later, as part of the Dementia Care Strategy, the government announced an expansion of this service. The idea is that there should be clinics all around the country, based in hospitals, in GP surgeries or on the high street, and that they should be 'one-stop shops' offering expert assessment, earlier diagnosis, support, information and advice to people with dementia and their families.

Memory clinics should be able to offer at least some of the following:

- an assessment of a person's problems and an accurate diagnosis;
- information about possible treatment;
- details of local support groups;
- 'carers' courses' to help carers deal with everyday management;
- information on counselling for patient and carer;
- practical help – for example, talks from lawyers on setting up Power of Attorney;
- research programmes in which people with dementia may be invited to take part.

Kate Dawson is a research nurse at the memory clinic at Addenbrooke's Hospital in Cambridge.

> Our clinic is held between 9 a.m. and 1 p.m. every Tuesday morning. At one time we were unique, but now there are other memory clinics in our area and elsewhere in major hospitals. There is generally more awareness of early-onset dementia. Patients are referred to us by GPs and consultants. When they arrive they are seen for a memory assessment by myself or a colleague, while a doctor talks to the carer on his or her own – although people with dementia and their carers are seen together too. We see six or seven new patients and the same number of follow-up patients every day, and have an

afternoon team meeting to work out the best way forward for each individual.

We are the first port of call for a second opinion, so many of those who come here have either not been diagnosed or their diagnosis is uncertain. We organize investigations and go through them so that a diagnosis can be made.

Then I will talk to carers about support in the community. Some don't want the information at that point so I tell them they can always come back to us in the future. Others want someone to talk to or to visit them at home. We have an early-onset dementia nurse in the community here as there are different issues to consider for younger people, including ensuring that they are 'medically retired' from work rather than made redundant.

Some are prescribed the appropriate drugs, and if that's the case we will follow them up. We work with older people too but they tend to be referred to old-age psychiatrists. Younger people don't have that route. We also let them know if there are any clinical trials, which many are keen to take part in.

Specialist support groups

Some of the rarer forms of dementia, for example Pick's disease, seem especially to affect younger people. Both national and local support groups have been set up to offer those with the condition and their carers the opportunity to discover more about the illness and its management.

The Pick's Disease Support Group (contact details on p. 110) says that there are relatively few facilities for younger people, and those which do exist are not always appropriate for those with fronto-temporal dementias, including Pick's. These are a group of rare disorders mostly affecting the frontal and anterior temporal lobes of the brain, and often causing different symptoms – for example, personality changes – rather than memory loss, as with Alzheimer's and the better-known dementias.

The Group offers help for those with Pick's, Lewy body dementia, frontal lobe degeneration and primary progressive aphasia. Log on to its website and you will find information on these dementias and the research that is being done into causes and cures. There are practical tips on day-to-day management, regional contacts, newsletters and information about meetings and seminars. There is also an online membership forum.

'We find value in talking with one another about the challenges we face as care-givers and the changes we see in our loved ones,' says one member.

The Huntington's Disease Association (HDA; contact details on p. 109) supports all those affected by Huntington's, also their families, friends and healthcare professionals. The HDA has teams of regional care advisers who provide information and advice, give talks and can advise on issues such as respite and residential care.

There are local branches and groups where families and carers can share experiences, and the group also raises funds for research. The Association produces fact-sheets about Huntington's and there is an online message board forum for members.

The CJD Support Network (contact details on p. 108) was set up in 1995 by relatives of some of the young people affected by Creutzfeldt-Jakob disease, to support those with the condition, carers and health professionals. They produce information sheets on the different forms of CJD and a newsletter, as well as promoting quality care for those affected, campaigning and promoting research.

Practical and emotional support is offered, including support for those who are at higher risk of developing CJD through blood transfusions or the use of surgical instruments (for more about this see p. 6). The Network can offer grants for families in need and can link families to other local carers for mutual support if required.

The Clive Project (contact details on p. 108) is an Oxfordshire-based service for younger people with all types of dementia, their families and friends. Their aim is to help individuals and their families live life to the full, whatever their diagnosis.

The Project was named for Clive Beaumont, an army officer who developed early-onset dementia when he was only in his forties and had two very small children. Sadly, Clive died in 1999 aged 51, but his name lives on in the form of this support organization. Among the kinds of help the project offers are a one-to-one support service where the person with dementia is 'partnered' with a trained support worker who works out an individualized programme of activities for between two and four hours a week. The Project's family support service offers both individual and group support, discussions and information, social events and contacts, and a newsletter. There's a club which runs social events and an evening café where people with dementia and carers can meet once a month.

'Let's get dementia out of the shadows,' says one member.

Other organizations such as the Multiple Sclerosis Society and Parkinson's UK can also offer help and support where appropriate.

Admiral nurses

Most people will have heard of Macmillan nurses, who specialize in the care of people with cancer. Admiral nurses, who are mental-health nurses specializing in dementia care, can offer help to people of any age with dementia and their carers. At present there isn't an Admiral nursing service all over the country, but you can obtain help and advice from Admiral Nursing DIRECT, their national helpline (contact details on p. 107).

Ian Weatherhead is a registered mental-health nurse who became an Admiral nurse because he wanted the challenge of working with families as well as people with dementia themselves.

There are more than 80 of us around the country now, and families can refer themselves, call the Admiral Nursing DIRECT helpline, or be referred by their GP or local mental-health team. Initially I will go and see the families or carers, with or without the person they're caring for being present. I talk to them and do an assessment of the family's needs, giving them the opportunity to tell me about the stress of caring and also the satisfaction it can bring, because it isn't all negative! Then we come to a mutual agreement about what is needed to make everyone's life easier. If the family are struggling, I will see them regularly for weeks or months, or perhaps less often as their confidence improves. Sometimes, a one-off visit, offering help and advice on something like claiming benefits or coping with difficult behaviour, is all that is needed. With other families, I will be there right through from initial diagnosis to end-of-life. We can also offer advice on things like home care or respite care for families.

If there's no Admiral nurse in their areas, families can call our helpline, which is staffed by Admiral nurses, and get answers to specific questions, advice and support.

Dementia UK (contact details on p. 108) is the national charity set up in the 1980s to improve the quality of life for people with dementia. They work in partnership with the NHS and other interested organizations to promote and develop Admiral nursing, as well as establishing a national network of carers, families and friends of people with dementia, and providing appropriate training for care staff and other health professionals.

6

Practical matters

Being given a diagnosis of early-onset dementia will, of course, have a huge emotional impact – but there are practical matters which also need to be considered. At first it is likely that it will all go round and round in your head. What will happen about work? Can we afford to go on living in this house? What benefits are available to help us? Can I continue to drive? Whether you are the one with dementia or the carer, there's a lot you will need to find out. It can be reassuring to know that there is help out there and that the various support groups for people with dementia can offer advice on all these practical issues.

Work

Depending how long it has taken you to obtain an accurate diagnosis, and also depending on the job you do, it may be possible for you to continue working even after you have found out you have dementia. Your employers may have noticed that you are struggling and some can be surprisingly understanding, though attitudes do vary.

Peter was a driver with London Underground when he was diagnosed with early-onset Alzheimer's in his early fifties.

They were very good when I told them about my diagnosis, though it was new ground for them and I felt like something of a pioneer. I told the human resources manager and she took a break to consider my situation.

She came back to tell me I could continue as a driver for the time being, but that every six months I would be assessed by an 'instructor operator' to make sure I was still able to do the job. This continued for eighteen months, but then I decided for myself that I couldn't carry on. I carried around with me the nightmare of getting sacked for doing something wrong and I decided it was time for me to leave.

I was pleasantly surprised by my colleagues' attitudes as well. Everyone – both male and female – was extremely sympathetic and helpful. As for money, my wife has always been better at handling the family finances than I was and she just took over more and more, which I was quite happy to let her do.

Cyril, a former maintenance manager for a training college, was less fortunate. When his dementia was diagnosed he was offered a choice between a cleaning job and early retirement. Unfortunately he and his wife lived in college accommodation, so losing his job meant the couple losing their home as well. Cyril's wife, Patricia, says,

We were on the council waiting list, but all they could offer was a private flat where the landlord wouldn't allow us to keep our much-loved dog. It was extremely stressful until Cyril's mother died and we were able, with his brother's agreement, to move back into the family home, although this did mean us leaving all our friends and family behind.

It is, of course, vital to be honest with your manager, boss or human resources department about your situation, showing them your medical reports if necessary. Far better to tell them what is wrong and what you are having difficulty with, rather than leaving them to find out for themselves after there have been complaints or you have made (possibly expensive) mistakes. Discuss the risks and responsibilities of your present job with the relevant people and try to decide together whether you are able to carry on working. Are you still capable of doing your original job? Could you be transferred to a part-time position? Might there perhaps be something less demanding you could do, within the same organization?

If you have to give up work, you will need to negotiate retirement due to sickness or early retirement with your boss. Companies are supposed to make 'reasonable adjustments' to accommodate disabled workers within the ordinary workforce under the Disability Discrimination Act (DDA) of 1995. The DDA defines 'disability' as 'a physical or mental impairment which has a substantial or long-term adverse effect on an employee's ability to carry out normal day-to-day activities'.

Impairments, it should be noted, don't just include lack of mobility, eyesight and hearing – the obvious physical difficulties – but also things like memory and the ability to concentrate, learn and understand, all of which may affect someone with dementia. The Equality and Human Rights Commission website (contact details on p. 109) has useful information about your rights under this Act. Your trade union representative will be able to help you negotiate a fair settlement, and it's worth remembering that some unions have benevolent or hardship funds which give grants or other support to members who are unable to carry on with their normal work.

Debt problems are unfortunately common among families where a breadwinner is diagnosed with early-onset dementia. Independent advice is available from the National Debtline (contact details on p. 109).

John and Pamela found that setting up an IVA (individual voluntary arrangement) helped with their money difficulties. John says,

> I was on sick pay while I was being diagnosed. After a couple of months my employer began asking questions. Once I told them I had Pick's disease and gave them some information about it they were very sympathetic and helped all they could.
>
> Unfortunately because of the illness I had run up huge debts on credit cards as well as losing my income. Pamela, who is now the family breadwinner, set up an IVA, but we still get letters from debt companies.

In an era of high unemployment it may be hard for you to find another job, but it is worth discussing your options with the Disability Employment Adviser and the nearest Jobcentre Plus. So much depends on what kind of dementia you have and how it affects you. As we have already seen, it is a very individual condition, especially in its early stages. If you can't continue with your previous job, there may be something else you can do that uses some of your remaining skills.

Voluntary work – possibly for one of the dementia charities – is another possibility.

Giving up paid work before you reach pension age will affect your right to a state pension, but you can protect this by claiming National Insurance credits. This is a complex procedure: to find out more about organizing it, contact the Alzheimer's Society or your local Citizens Advice office.

Benefits

People living with dementia and their carers are entitled to financial help from the state. Some of this is means-tested – i.e. it depends how much you are earning or how much National Insurance you have paid over the years – and some is non-means-tested and can be claimed according to need. You can apply online at <www.dwp.gov.uk> or call the Benefits Enquiry Line on 0800 88 22 00 for more information.

As anyone who has ever claimed any kind of benefit knows, finding your way through the thickets of bureaucracy, discovering what you are entitled to and actually getting it is not always straightforward. There is a lot of form-filling and you may be asked the same questions over and over again. However, it is always worth persevering, and also worth remembering that you are *entitled* to this help – no-one is doing you a favour. The social security system was invented to help those who, through no fault of their own, have fallen on hard times because of injury or illness. That means you, so don't be afraid to claim what is yours.

Tony is a former journalist who was diagnosed with early-onset Alzheimer's six years ago. It took him five years to get a diagnosis.

The quality of my work deteriorated and eventually I lost my job. My GP was not very helpful and put it down to stress. I would wake up in the morning not knowing where I was and thought I was going mad. I did see a psychiatrist but the medication he gave me didn't help. Eventually I was referred to a neurologist, and after two MRI scans I got my diagnosis, which was devastating. I didn't even know Alzheimer's could affect younger people.

Once I knew what was wrong I became quite militant about wanting to know what help was out there and how I was going to live. I was means-tested by the Department of Work and Pensions, and with the help of my neurologist managed to get Disability Living Allowance, Incapacity Benefit, Income Support and help with housing costs and Council Tax. It does seem to be a lottery, depending how determined you are.

The main benefit for people below retirement age who are disabled is called Disability Living Allowance, or DLA. DLA is payable to anyone under 65 who needs help either with personal care or with mobility. There are three different rates of the 'personal care' component, and two different rates of the 'mobility' component, and these are assessed according to individual need. DLA is paid out tax-free and is non-means-tested. It doesn't depend on your income, your savings, if any, or your National Insurance contributions.

Not surprisingly, the forms you have to fill in to claim DLA are long and complicated, and in order to get the amount of money you're entitled to it's important to make the appropriate claims. Don't let pride stop you from asking for the help you need. If there are things you can't do without help, or you need supervision because of memory problems, then say so. Get advice from one of the disability support groups or Citizens Advice on filling in the forms.

The top rate of the 'care' component of DLA is paid to those who need considerable help and support to do everyday things like wash, dress, go to the toilet, prepare and eat meals, and take medication. Someone with dementia who needs regular supervision day and/or night to stop him or her wandering away, leaving the gas on or otherwise getting into danger, should also be eligible for the top rate.

Someone who needs less help might be eligible for the middle rate of DLA, and someone who needs just a little supervision – perhaps with preparing a cooked meal – may be eligible for the lower rate. However, this all depends very much on individual needs, and when filling in the forms you should be sure to include everything with which you need help.

The 'mobility' component is paid out at a higher rate to people who can't walk, or whose walking is very difficult because of pain, stiffness or weakness. A lower rate may be paid to those whose dementia means that they need to be supervised when going anywhere because they might get lost, be unable to find their way around or are inclined to wander off. Again, the claims are all judged on an individual basis, and if the person claiming becomes sicker or more disabled, a higher rate of benefit should be claimed.

Statutory sick pay is payable by employers for up to 28 weeks in any period of sickness. The person to whom it is paid must be earning a certain amount every week and must be unable to work. This benefit is taxable.

Employment and Support Allowance is a new benefit that was introduced in 2008 to replace Incapacity Benefit and Income Support (if claimed because of disability). In order to claim this you must have been working and have paid National Insurance contributions, and you will be assessed on your current ability to work. You'll need to provide medical evidence of your inability to work.

Other benefits you may be able to claim include Income Support, which is payable to people under 60 with low incomes and limited savings; Jobseeker's Allowance, if you are capable of and actively seeking work; Housing Benefit, to help with the cost of housing; Council Tax Benefit, to reduce the amount of Council Tax you have to pay – your local authority will be able to tell you about this. Some of these benefits are means-tested and some depend on your level of National Insurance contributions. Remember too that carers are entitled to benefits in their own right. We will be looking at the financial help available to them, usually through Carer's Allowance, in the next chapter.

Other payments may be made to those in special need. A Winter Fuel Payment is paid to everyone over 60, regardless of means, to help with the cost of gas and electricity over the winter. There is also a Social Fund which sometimes offers low-cost loans and grants in times of crisis. Once you are on benefits, some NHS treatments become cheap or free: for example, prescriptions, dental treatment, sight tests and hospital travel costs.

It is also worth knowing that there are charities and hardship funds which provide grants for those in special need, ranging from trade unions to small and little-known charities. SSAFA Forces Help (contact details on p. 110), for example, can offer support to serving and former military personnel and their families, as can ABF The Soldiers' Charity and the RAF Benevolent Fund (contact details on pp. 107 and 110, respectively). Elizabeth Finn Care (contact details on p. 109) offers grants to low-income families in need. Most occupations, from solicitors to gardeners and musicians, have benevolent funds which can help out former members of the profession who have fallen on hard times. Eligibility criteria vary but it is always worth checking. Much, of course, will depend on your personal circumstances, but there is help out there.

Driving

Driving can be a big issue for people diagnosed with early-onset dementia (and, indeed, for those diagnosed later in life). Unless you live in the centre of a major city, having access to your own transport is often felt to be essential. Being a driver enables you to go where you want, when you want, and even those of us who are keen to cut down our carbon emissions and save the planet often find that managing without a car, and relying on public transport, is just too complicated and inconvenient.

Being diagnosed with dementia does not automatically mean you have to give up driving immediately. In the early stages of your illness, you may be able to manage quite well. You may retain your existing driving skills, especially if you stick to familiar routes and have someone with you in the car to help with navigating. However, eventually the time will come when you are no longer safe on the road. You may recognize that time yourself and feel increasingly nervous and uncomfortable at the wheel. If you have never been enthusiastic about driving, the time to give up could come sooner rather than later.

If you have been driving for many years you probably do it almost automatically. However, driving is a complex skill which involves co-ordinating several different physical actions and thought processes. You need to control the car, read road signs, be aware of other road users, both motorists and pedestrians, be able to anticipate possible problems, find your way about and avoid accidents. Some people lose confidence in their driving abilities as they get older, even without the added complication of dementia.

If you have been diagnosed with dementia and you want to go on driving, you should inform the DVLA (contact details on p. 108). They will send you a questionnaire asking permission for them to contact your medical team to work out whether or not you are still fit to drive, and may ask you to take a 'driving assessment'. (You can choose to do this on your own initiative if you are beginning to feel unsure about driving.)

If the DVLA decide you are still fit to drive they will issue you with a new driving licence which is usually valid for a year, after which your condition should be reviewed. If you are considered no longer fit to drive, you have to return your licence to the DVLA. There is an appeals process if you disagree with the DVLA's decision.

A person with dementia who did not inform the DVLA about the diagnosis, or who continued to drive after the DVLA had decided he or she was no longer safe on the road, would be breaking the law. It is also essential to tell your insurance company you have dementia as your insurance could become invalid if you did not disclose your illness. Again, it is against the law to drive without valid insurance.

If you are a partner or carer, it's a good idea to monitor the person's driving and make sure your loved one's condition is not deteriorating so quickly that he or she is not safe on the roads. You can inform the DVLA and ask them for a medical assessment if you have concerns about the person's driving ability. It is worth remembering that medication – for example, sleeping tablets or anti-depressants – can sometimes affect the ability to drive. Obtain medical advice if this seems to be the case.

It can be very distressing for someone with dementia to be told he or she is no longer able to drive, especially if driving has been relied upon for work and social life for many years. Partners, carers, friends and family members should be ready to listen, sympathize and help the person with dementia to reorganize life as far as possible using taxis and public transport instead of the car, or to get used to being a passenger rather than a driver. The Alzheimer's Society recommends involving the person in making the new arrangements as far as possible, as well as pointing out the advantages of being a car-free household – no road tax, expensive garage bills or parking charges to pay, for example! Shopping and banking can be done online and short journeys can be done on foot, providing the beginnings of an exercise routine. If there are still drivers in the family, joining a 'car club', where you pay an annual subscription and then a small fee when you really *need* to use a car, can be an economical alternative for the whole family.

Occasionally someone with dementia may refuse to give up driving, even on medical advice, and simply not understand that he or she is no longer safe on the road. This is, of course, extremely upsetting for all concerned. Support groups may be able to suggest solutions as other families may have had to face the same problem.

Travelling and holidays

Just because someone with dementia is no longer able to drive should not mean needing to miss out on the pleasure and relaxation of a holiday. In fact, it may be even *more* important that both the person and the carer have 'time off' away from normal routines while the person with dementia is still able to enjoy a break.

Andrew, Laura's husband and main carer, says,

Laura has lost a lot of her skills since she was diagnosed with Alzheimer's. She can't complete a conversation, dress herself properly, cook or find her way around, but she is very fit physically – much fitter than I am – and she does love her holidays.

With the help of our children, who sometimes travel with us, we have been on mountain walking holidays, skiing and a couple of cruises, and Laura loves them. She never was one to sit around doing nothing and that hasn't changed. I hobble along and she strides out in front. When we go on cruises she likes to get off the ship and see something. I do have to keep an eye on her all the time – she once had her purse stolen – but I can't put a ball and chain on her and I wouldn't want to try. She still has some concept of the future and understands when I tell her we are going on holiday and she still gets excited. I would hate to deprive her of that.

Some people with dementia are soothed by everyday routine and find being in unfamiliar places distressing and confusing. This is more common in the later stages of the illness, but clearly if the person you're caring for is happier on home ground, then holidays may not be appropriate for him or her (though you should still be able to take a break if you are a carer!).

It's always important to choose the right holiday, and especially so if you or anyone in the party has special needs. The Disability Discrimination Act of 1995 was intended to remove any physical barriers and enable those with special needs to enjoy the same breaks as everyone else. Nor are companies permitted to charge more for accessibility. Of course, the Act only applies to holiday facilities in the UK, but most holiday companies will try to accommodate customers with special needs as long as you make it clear when booking exactly what will be required.

Check with your holiday company or airline what help they can provide. If you choose to travel by train, check out the Assisted Passenger Reservation Service for train travel in the UK and via Eurostar. Two days' notice before travelling is required but it is, of course, preferable to make your plans well in advance. When arranging travel insurance, check that any health policy you take out covers 'pre-existing conditions'. Always be open and honest about what you, as carer, and the person with dementia need.

If you are concerned about your loved one wandering off and getting lost – which can easily happen in a crowded airport or resort – make sure he or she is wearing a MedicAlert pendant or bracelet. These have details of the medical condition engraved on them, and also emergency numbers to call. More information from MedicAlert on 0800 581 420 or <www.medicalert.org.uk>. The Pick's Disease Support Group produces awareness cards which you or the person affected can carry, explaining possible memory or behaviour problems.

If you are travelling within Europe you should obtain a European Health Insurance Card (EHIC) which replaces the old E111 insurance form. This entitles you to medical care on the same basis as the nationals of the country you're travelling to. Be warned, however: you may have to pay up front and then claim the costs back if that's the usual procedure in the country you are in. The EHIC lasts for five years and does include treatment for pre-existing medical conditions. Call 0845 606 2030 or look at the website <www.ehic.org.uk> for more information.

There are many travel companies which specialize in providing holidays for people with disabilities, including dementia. Vitalise (contact details on p. 111) is a long-established charity offering holiday breaks in five centres in the UK for those with disabilities. Their holidays include specially organized weeks for people with dementia and their carers. Because there are staff on hand to offer support, carers do get time to themselves on these breaks.

Other organizations focusing more on those with physical disabilities, but worth checking out to see what they have to offer, include Tourism for All (contact details on p. 111) which has comprehensive information on UK travel for those with disabilities and also some information about travelling abroad. Enable Holidays (contact details on p. 109) organize holidays in Europe and the USA for wheelchair users and others with limited mobility, but say they also want to help people with a 'wider range of disabilities to enjoy holidays abroad'.

Making life easier

A wide variety of gadgets and gizmos is available to help people with disabilities to cope with everyday life. Some are obviously geared towards people with mobility problems or sight or hearing difficulties, but others can help with memory, thought processes and understanding – so-called 'cognitive' problems such as those experienced by those with dementia. Some are very low-tech – pinboards, diaries, calendars, clocks and photographs which can serve as memory aids for those who would benefit from them. Organizations like the Disabled Living Foundation (contact details on p. 108) have information about what is available if the problems experienced are more physical.

There are also commercial companies such as Hearing and Mobility (contact details on p. 109) selling aids to daily living.

The term used to describe systems and devices that help people to do things they wouldn't otherwise be able to do is 'assistive technology', and this can cover anything from diaries and notebooks to sophisticated electronic monitors, similar to satnavs, which enable carers to track loved ones who may wander or get lost. Some of these may be appropriate for some people with dementia, depending on their symptoms, level of understanding and personal preferences.

Becoming very forgetful or being unable to remember basic skills like cooking or making a cup of tea can have safety implications, and this can be frightening for both people with dementia and their carers and families. Leaving the gas on or a kettle to boil dry, running a bath and then forgetting about it and the resulting flood, wandering or becoming confused about the medication prescribed, can all be sources of great worry for carers and lead to people with dementia having to be admitted to residential care before they otherwise would. Assistive technology, used wisely, can mean a better and more independent quality of life for the person and peace of mind for the carer.

The AT Dementia website (contact details on p. 107) is especially useful as it divides the products available into four categories:

- prompts and reminders, including clocks and calendar clocks; 'memo minders' which play a pre-recorded message when the person walks past with a reminder to do or not do something; medication reminders with audible or visual alerts; and item locator devices to help find lost keys or anything that has been misplaced;
- communication devices, such as telephones with pre-programmable numbers and spaces for photos of friends and relatives, and message boards to aid communication;

- leisure activities – things like easy-to-use computer keyboards, TV and radio remote controls, computer games, talking photograph albums and other reminiscence materials;
- safety – smoke and carbon monoxide alarms, gas and flood detectors, pagers, automatic lights, and sophisticated sensor equipment which can monitor someone's whereabouts and activities and alert carers or a monitoring centre if there may be a problem.

The website also explains how best to choose appropriate products and how they are installed and maintained.

Planning for the future

Many people diagnosed with early-onset dementia feel that the best way to cope is to live from day to day and make the most of the time you have left with your loved ones. However, it is also important to face the fact that dementia is a progressive condition and that you will not always be as well as you are at the time of diagnosis. There are some practical steps you should take at this stage to make sure that your family is protected and that your wishes are carried out when you are no longer able to make decisions for yourself.

The Mental Capacity Act 2005 states that people can choose someone to manage their affairs – which means finances, property and personal welfare – when they no longer can, through what is known as a Lasting Power of Attorney or LPA. Once a person has lost the capacity to make decisions for him- or herself, a different process must be followed, so it is really better to plan ahead.

An LPA is a legal document which allows you to appoint another person to act on your behalf. This person – the 'attorney' – must be over 18, and the LPA must be registered with the Office of the Public Guardian (contact details on p. 110), which can send out an application pack on request.

There are two different kinds of LPA. One is for matters related to property and business – for example writing cheques, paying bills and selling property. The 'attorney' can make decisions about these matters whether or not the person with dementia still has capacity him- or herself. The other kind of LPA relates to personal welfare and covers things like making decisions about what kind of medical treatment the person with dementia does or does not receive, and whether that person should be in residential care and, if so, where. These decisions can only be made by the 'attorney' once the person with dementia has lost the capacity to make them him- or herself.

You can see that setting up an LPA involves a lot of important decisions. If you need advice on what is best, you might like to consult a solicitor who has experience in this area. The Law Society (contact details on p. 109) should be able to put you in touch with someone appropriate and the Alzheimer's Society can also offer advice.

You might also consider seeing a solicitor if your financial affairs are at all complex, for instance if you own a lot of property and need to set up trusts to manage your assets. If you have not made a will, it's essential that you do so now. If you don't, your 'estate' – everything you own when you die – may not be distributed as you would wish. You might also like to consider signing a 'Living Will' or 'Advance Directive' which states clearly what medical treatments you would want to be given or withheld if you became terminally ill and were incapable of making your wishes known at the time. The Natural Death Centre (contact details on p. 110) can give you information about this.

While you are relatively fit and well, you can make life easier and less complicated by, for example, arranging for bills to be paid by direct debit or standing order, and for pensions and benefits to be paid directly into your bank account. It can help to write down everything you have paid in or taken out in a simple cash book. Remember to include money you have taken out of cash machines. If you would like a relative, close friend or carer to manage your bank account for you, you can ask your bank for a 'third party mandate' which enables someone to do this.

If you have set up an LPA it is recommended that you and your 'attorney' should have separate rather than joint bank accounts, in case you need to be means-tested if you need residential care as your illness progresses.

If you own your home – either on your own or jointly with a partner – it might be advisable to tell the mortgage company about your change of circumstances, and think carefully about whether you can afford to carry on paying the mortgage on a reduced income, or whether moving to a smaller, cheaper property might be your best option.

If, at a later date, you need to move into a care home, it is worth remembering that you do not have to sell your home to pay for care if your husband, wife or unmarried partner, a close relative over 60 or under 16, a carer or close relative under 60 who is incapacitated, needs to go on living there. However, the rules about paying for care are complicated and changing all the time, so it's best to get legal advice from your local Citizens Advice office, the Alzheimer's Society or organizations such as Age UK (contact details on p. 107).

7

Carers and families

The impact of early-onset dementia on partners and families can't be overestimated. Any serious illness has huge repercussions for families, of course, but there is something uniquely devastating about seeing the person you loved and knew so well becoming a virtual stranger. No-one *chooses* to become a carer in these circumstances. Once you were husband and wife, lovers, partners and best friends – and now, slowly but inevitably, one of you is becoming that strange modern word, a 'carer', and the other is being cared for.

Una, whose husband was diagnosed with dementia in his mid-fifties, puts it this way:

> Caring creeps up on you and you gradually take on the role without really realizing it. Jim could manage quite well at first but I found myself doing more and more for him, which was frustrating for him and heartbreaking for me. When I look back now I'm sure I would have thought I couldn't cope with it all, but you do. You just do. I'm proud, now, to see Jim looking as well and smart as he always did – he is ex-army – and going for outings and walks, looking around and enjoying the life we share, even though he can't express what he's feeling. Knowing I have helped to make that happen is rewarding, even if it hasn't been easy.

Caring can be hard work. It can be difficult, frustrating and, as Una says, heartbreaking. As a carer – or a potential carer – there are two vital things you need to remember:

- You are not alone. There is a lot of help out there. You are entitled to it so make sure you get it!
- You matter, too. Caring for someone inevitably means some sacrifices on your part but it shouldn't mean sacrificing your entire life. It's easy to run yourself into the ground when you

are caring for someone, putting the other person's needs before your own, doing what you feel you 'ought' to do rather than what you want and need to do. As a carer, you have rights, and that includes the right to some life of your own. When you are thinking about how much caring you are able to do, you have to consider your partner's needs, yes, but also your own. You also have to consider your other commitments – to your children, perhaps to your parents, to your work. Whatever solutions you find need to work for you, all of you. This is not the time to worry about what other people might think!

Caring for the carers

It's only in the last few years that the rights of carers have been recognized. In the past it was simply assumed that anyone with a seriously ill or disabled family member would just 'get on with it' and do the best he or she could. Slowly, carers' voices began to be heard, thanks to organizations like Carers UK (contact details on p. 108), who point out the vast amount of unpaid caring work done in the UK, day after day, week after week. Without carers, the NHS or Social Services would have to increase their budgets by at least £87 *billion* to pay for care, and it's estimated that one in eight adults is a carer.

You may never have thought of yourself as a carer. After all, looking after your loved ones is just something you do, isn't it – part of your commitment to one another 'in sickness and in health' whether you are actually married or not? Even if your partner hasn't had an official diagnosis, if you're having to help him or her with what social workers call 'activities of daily living', you're a carer. You can help yourself by:

- including your wider family and friends in the caring;
- telling your GP so that he or she can monitor your health, as well as your partner's, and possibly direct you to other sources of help like local carers' groups;

- contacting some of the support organizations listed on pages 107–111 to find out what help they can offer;
- letting your employer know, if you are still working and want to continue. The Work and Families Act 2006 gave carers the right to request flexible working from their employer to accommodate their caring responsibilities;
- making sure you look after yourself (more about this later in this chapter!). You will be doing your partner no favours if you neglect your own well-being and become too exhausted and stressed to provide adequate care.

If you're new to caring, it can seem overwhelming and difficult to know where to start. Probably the best way is by contacting one of the three major carers' organizations, which have a vast amount of expertise at their disposal.

Carers UK (contact details on p. 108) can tell you everything you need to know about caring and they are also effective campaigners for carers' rights, so their website is a very good place to start. Whether your first concern is what to tell your employer, what to tell the children, how to involve Social Services or how you are going to cope financially, or you just need someone to talk to, they will be able to offer at least some of the answers.

Crossroads Care (contact details on p. 108) was named after the much-loved Midlands-based TV soap opera which was one of the first to feature a character who was a wheelchair user. They now provide practical support for carers and help around 35,000 people a year through local groups. Their help is very much user-led; they are very flexible and family-friendly, so whether you want to enquire about getting a break from caring or to be introduced to others in similar situations to your own, it is worth contacting them.

The Princess Royal Trust for Carers (contact details on p. 110) was set up in 1991 by HRH Princess Anne, and has lots of useful information including an online message board with tips for carers on any issues which arise through caring.

All the support charities for people with dementia, such as the Alzheimer's Society and the Pick's Disease Support Group, offer help to carers too.

Carers' benefits

As a carer you are entitled to help from the state on your own behalf, in addition to any benefits the person you're caring for might be claiming. The main financial benefit is the admittedly stingy Carer's Allowance. In 2009–10 this was set at a mere £53.20 per week if you were caring for at least 35 hours per week and not earning more than £95 a week from paid employment. This is obviously totally inadequate, and the House of Commons recommended in 2008 that it should be updated. All the carers' campaigning groups are working on this. However, it is there to be claimed.

You are also entitled to a carer's assessment from Social Services. This is in addition to the assessment given to the person you are caring for and is aimed at providing help for *you*, as a carer. You'll need to get in touch with the local Social Services, whose direct number will be listed in the phone book under the name of the local council, to ask for this assessment. Before you do so, and certainly before the social worker visits you to carry out the assessment, it's wise to sit down and think carefully about exactly what help you feel you need and what would make your life easier.

Carers UK have a lot of useful information to guide you through the assessment process and list some of the things the social worker will want to know so that the right help can be offered. It's a good idea to make some notes about these before the assessment takes place. For example:

- What do you actually have to do to help the person you're caring for – cooking, shopping, dealing with finances, giving personal care such as bathing and dressing and helping with eating?

- Does the person you're caring for have any physical disabilities in addition to the problems caused by the dementia? Would adaptations to your home (a shower instead of, or in addition to, a bath? a downstairs lavatory?) make life easier for both of you?
- What are the symptoms of the person with dementia, especially those you find particularly difficult to deal with – forgetfulness, aggression, difficult behaviour, incontinence, wandering?
- Do you have any health problems yourself?
- Are you able to sleep?
- Do you feel stressed or depressed some or all of the time?
- How many hours a week do you care for the person with dementia? Does anyone else help? For how long? Do you get regular or occasional breaks from caring?
- What sort of help would be most useful? This could be anything from someone to help with personal care on a regular basis to a break for the person with dementia at a day centre, night-time care, meals delivered, help with shopping, information about benefits and/or residential care, someone to talk to . . . (Not all these services will be available everywhere, and you may have to pay for some of them, but it is always worth asking.)
- Are you still working and do you want to carry on with your job?
- What other commitments do you have – for example, elderly parents or young children?

Try and give the social worker a realistic picture of your situation. This is not the time to be stoical and insist that you can continue to cope on your own when in reality you may be near breaking point. Caring for someone with early-onset dementia is a tough job, no matter how much you love them and how strong you are. If you feel angry, and resentful at having to become a full-time carer, then say so. You're a human being, not a plaster saint.

When you have had your assessment, Social Services have to draw up a care plan, taking into account your needs as a carer as well as the needs of your partner. Exactly how much help is offered, and what kind of help, depends on your circumstances and on where you live. You could be offered help with transport, details of support groups, respite care for the person with dementia to give you the chance of a break – a variety of types of help. You could also ask the social workers about Direct Payments, which is a system by which carers are given money to 'buy in' the help they need rather than having it provided directly by Social Services. This gives you more control about exactly what help you receive.

It doesn't cost you anything to get a carer's assessment but you may be asked to pay for some or all of the services offered, depending on your financial circumstances and the area you live in. You can ask how these charges are calculated and appeal if you feel they are unfair or that you are unable to pay. As your loved one's condition deteriorates, both your needs may change and you will probably need to contact Social Services again to access further help.

Dealing with feelings

There are always practical problems to sort out when you become a carer, but you will find that you are on an emotional roller-coaster too. The relationship you have with your partner, or with a close friend or family member if you're caring for someone other than a partner, is bound to change over the years. When once you were equal partners, sharing most things, helping one another out, depending on one another for sympathy, support and help with anything from fixing a leaking tap to deciding where to go on holiday, life is now very different and it can take a considerable time to adjust.

Relate, the relationships charity (contact details on p. 110), can offer face-to-face, email or telephone counselling to couples and individuals in this situation. They are aware that any serious illness, including dementia, can lead to the break-up of relationships, especially if there were difficulties between the couple before the illness took hold.

As one of their experienced counsellors says:

> The relationship inevitably becomes less equal when one of you is a carer and the other cared-for. Practical things need to change and this can cause resentment. With dementia, the changes may happen gradually so the two of you do have time to plan for the future. Sessions with a counsellor may help you work on your communication skills so that you can *talk* – expressing yourself in an open, honest, non-confrontational way – and *listen*, hearing the emotions as well as the words. The illness almost becomes a third party in the relationship and it's OK to feel angry with it.
>
> It helps to think creatively and give the ill person some responsibilities, so he or she is not just being cared for. Breaks and respite care are important too. Both carer and cared-for may be glad to see the back of one another from time to time!

Especially as your partner's condition worsens, you may find your feelings for him or her change in ways you had not expected, and this can be distressing. You may have loved this person for many years but suddenly feel you can't bear to be in his or her company any longer. This isn't, after all, the man or woman you fell in love with, but a childish, aggressive or indifferent stranger. It's absolutely natural that you sometimes feel anger and resentment or even 'why did this have to happen to us?'

Mixed with this are other, conflicting emotions – love, pity, sympathy and guilt. It's not your loved one's fault that he or she has developed dementia, after all. Thinking of the dynamic, humorous, gentle or fun person that once was, and then comparing that image with the person you now care for, can tear your heart out.

You are having to deal with grief and loss, even though your loved one is still alive and still with you. You have lost your best friend, your lover, your co-parent. You have lost the future you planned to share, all the things you thought you would do together 'when the kids leave home' or 'when I (or we) retire'. Inevitably you have lost – or will soon lose – part of your social life, as some friends and acquaintances are unable to cope with the new state of affairs and drift away. A more limited income will probably mean you have to cut back on some of the activities you used to enjoy. It's a lot to take in.

Let yourself grieve. Where feelings and emotions are concerned, there is no 'right' or 'wrong' way to feel. Whether you feel angry, sad, resentful, guilty or anything else, you are entitled to your feelings. Acknowledge them. If you have brought up a family, think back to your children's babyhood. Much as you loved them, there were almost certainly times – at three in the morning when the baby wouldn't sleep, on wet winter Sundays when the toddler demanded to hear that nursery rhyme CD for the umpteenth time – when you felt like walking out. That sort of exasperation is entirely natural, so don't feel guilty about it. When you're tempted to snap at your partner, take a deep breath and go into another room, punch a cushion, make faces at yourself in a mirror or call one of the friends you have (hopefully) made at the carers' group. They will have been there too.

The impact of a condition like dementia on a couple's sex life is something that isn't often talked about. As your relationship changes from an equal partnership to one of carer and cared-for, the intimate side of the relationship is bound to change too. Sex is not equally important to all couples, but it's an aspect of loving that may be hard to lose.

In its early stages, early-onset dementia does not have to mean the end of your sex life; physical closeness can be very comforting and life-affirming at a time of great change. As the disease progresses, the partner with dementia might lose interest in sex, be unable or unwilling to 'perform', or become *more* interested and more demanding. Personality changes might lead to aggressive or uncaring behaviour in a partner who was previously tender and caring. This is, of course, terribly distressing for the other partner. Some people with more advanced dementia, as we have seen, behave inappropriately, making sexual advances to strangers, perhaps because they want to be hugged or because they mistake the stranger for a loved partner. The Alzheimer's Society can offer help for this kind of problem, and you might also benefit from counselling or a frank discussion with your partner's GP or consultant. As carer, you might feel just as loving towards your partner – or you might feel that sex is no longer appropriate. In either case you can be certain you are not alone. Other carers will have been through similar, or the same, emotions and it can help to talk it over, perhaps on one of the online forums where you can be anonymous if you choose. It can also help to remember that the problem is caused by the illness, not by your partner.

The value of carers' groups and organizations offering support to those with early-onset dementia and their families lies in the knowledge that others really do understand what you are going through. If you really feel you are coming to the end of your tether, then see about getting some counselling yourself. Your GP will be able to refer you for NHS help, or you can get in touch with the British Association for Counselling and Psychotherapy (contact details on p. 107). They have an online directory of counsellors and psychotherapists which you can search by region to find someone in your area who can help.

Don't forget, either, that the befriending charity Samaritans are there 24/7 to offer a listening ear: 08457 90 90 90.

Looking after yourself

A healthy lifestyle is vitally important for you as well as your partner. Good food, exercise, fresh air and sound sleep will help you to cope with caring and may also be things you and your partner can still share.

If you're one of the 20 per cent of British women or 25 per cent of British men who are still smoking – perhaps because you think it helps you cope with stress – do at least consider giving up. It's the best thing you can do for your health, and with help from nicotine replacement therapy and perhaps a local 'stop smoking' support group it need not be too painful. Contact the NHS Free Smoking Helpline (contact details on p. 110) for more information.

Advice on healthy eating is widely available and doesn't mean a lot of overpriced 'health' food, endless supplements or fad diets. A sensible balanced diet low in saturated fats and containing foods from all the major food groups, plenty of fruit and vegetables, with cakes, sweets and takeaways reserved for occasional treats, will keep you fit and stop excess pounds piling on. Make sure you are within the 'healthy weight' range for your height. Obesity levels in Britain have more than doubled since 1980, causing health professionals a great deal of concern as obesity is a risk factor for most serious illnesses, from diabetes to heart disease.

From a health point of view, it is worth checking your waist size. Women with a waist measurement of more than 35 inches (89 cm) are at high risk of health problems, as are men with a waist measurement of more than 40 inches (102 cm). Apple shapes – which means those who store fat around their waists – are more at risk of health problems than pear shapes, who store fat around their hips and thighs.

Both you and your partner will benefit from a healthy diet, and it has never been easier to adapt your eating patterns to a healthier version. Use semi-skimmed milk instead of full-fat, low-fat versions of things like cheese and yoghurt, low-fat spread instead of butter (or simply spread your butter more thinly). Grill instead of frying, trim the excess fat off meat, and replace puddings with fresh fruit.

Exercise, too, can benefit both you and your partner. Someone with dementia who has always enjoyed sport or outdoor exercise may still be able to do so. Walking, running, swimming, tennis, bowls, golf or keep-fit exercises can be enjoyed by both of you. If you haven't exercised before, why not just try to incorporate more walking into your everyday life? This might be particularly important if your partner has had to give up driving, or is planning to do so. Walking to the bus stop, the local shops or the train station can often provide the minimum of 30 minutes' exercise a day which experts recommend for keeping fit. Use the stairs instead of an escalator or lift, or get off the bus a stop or two earlier, and you will find you're getting fitter without having to join a gym or buy a pair of expensive trainers.

If you're having trouble sleeping, perhaps because you're worried about your partner getting up and wandering in the night, do see your GP. Sleeping tablets are often helpful in the short term, and he or she may also be able to recommend strategies which don't involve medication. A regular bedtime routine – both for you and for the person you care for – is important: a warm bath, the traditional milky drink and some undemanding TV or relaxing music can help, as can herbal remedies like lavender or valerian.

You also need relaxation time, which is why respite care and someone to share the caring is so vital. When you do get 'time off', make sure you use it wisely rather than rushing round trying to fit in everything you don't have time for when your partner is around. Consider taking up one of the 'relaxing' therapies such as yoga, meditation or autogenic training. (See Chapter 8 for more information about these.) Or it could be that a glass of wine, a box of chocolates and a good book, a session in the garden or a game of golf or snooker is just what you need to 'switch off' for a couple of hours. This is not an indulgence, it's a necessity. Don't feel guilty about taking a break.

Children

One of the saddest things about early-onset dementia is that many of the people affected may still have young children. People in their forties and fifties may, of course, already be grandparents, and with the trend to older parenthood and increasing numbers of second marriages, more children than ever before will come into contact with close relatives who have dementia.

In the past, children were often shielded from the truth about illness and it was genuinely thought better for them not to be told that a family member was seriously ill with something like cancer. These days, families are advised to share the information they have, even with quite small children, tailoring any explanation to the child's age and level of understanding.

This is because even quite small children will often be aware that something is wrong. If they are told nothing, they may become very anxious and insecure and even blame themselves, without understanding just what is happening. They may see a parent's or grandparent's behaviour change to something they don't recognize; they may see their other parent or siblings become distressed and preoccupied and seem no longer to have much time for them. In these circumstances it's far better for them to be told what is wrong, that Dad or Grandad has an illness which may make him behave in a way that might frighten, worry or upset them. Younger children need lots of reassurance that what has happened is *not* their fault, that Dad didn't get ill because they were naughty or said or did something 'wrong'.

The best thing carers – and indeed people with dementia themselves – can do is talk it over with their children and grand-children and make sure they know that they are still loved and that any problems, such as aggression, forgetfulness or embar-rassing behaviour, are a result of the illness and are not directed at them. Once children know what is happening, they can be surprisingly resilient and also caring. Organizations like the Princess Royal Trust, and others, run young carers' groups where youngsters can meet others who are in similar circumstances to themselves.

Encourage the children to tell you how they feel. Perhaps they are embarrassed if their friends come round, or they are being teased or bullied at school. If they are armed with simple explanations like 'my dad has a brain disease' they can explain to their friends. If they are being bullied, their school should be told. In fact, as with any family crisis, it's a good idea to tell the school so that allowances can be made for any behavioural changes caused by anxiety and worry.

A parent or grandparent with dementia may still enjoy the children's company, and familiar routines like walks or games in the garden or park should be kept up. Older children can accom-pany Dad or Grandad to the local shops and guide him in the right direction if he gets lost. As the condition worsens, carers will probably need to explain to the children that the important thing is that Dad or Grandad still needs to feel loved and cared for, even though he doesn't always remember their names.

Most literature for and about children and dementia focuses on the grandparent relationship, as this is, of course, most common. The Alzheimer's Society has a booklet, *Managing Together, Keeping Connected* about young children and grand-parents with dementia, which might be useful. The Mental Health Foundation (contact details on p. 109) publishes a book called *The Milk's in the Oven* which explains what dementia is and was specially written for children and young people.

8

Complementary medicine

When someone you love is diagnosed with a condition such as early-onset dementia, for which medical science can provide no cure, it's tempting to look beyond orthodox science for help. Surely there must be *some* way of treating this awful disease, something that can help?

Unfortunately that kind of desperation can easily make you prey to charlatans, who will promise miracle cures, take your money and run. Not that every complementary or 'alternative' practitioner is a charlatan, by any means. However, anyone looking at any kind of alternative treatment needs to be aware that they exist and that they are willing to exploit the vulnerable.

Having said that, many complementary therapies are well established and controlled by their own regulatory bodies, such as the National Institute of Medical Herbalists. If you are interested in exploring the 'complementary' route, do make sure that everyone you consult is a qualified member of the appropriate organization. It is also important to note that most complementary therapies do not have the wealth of scientific research behind them that pharmaceutical products do. Research into the efficacy of 'alternatives' tends to be sketchy and doesn't involve the years of double-blind, placebo-controlled clinical trials that conventional medicines have to go through before being marketed to the public.

Those who use complementary therapies say that scientific studies are replaced by years of experience and observation – about 3,000 years in the case of traditional Chinese medicine, for instance – and that there is at least *some* evidence that these therapies can help. Sceptics say that any perceived improvement is caused by the 'placebo' effect, which states that if you believe a treatment is going to do you good, then it probably will – but then, if you find it works for you, does that matter? And there is already a small amount of evidence that some therapies, at least, can be useful in reducing disturbed behaviour in people with dementia, calming them, and helping them to sleep. Relaxation techniques such as yoga, meditation and autogenic training can also help to reduce stress in carers and families.

Another important point is that although 'natural' remedies can sound more appealing as a way to treat dementia than prescribed drugs, just because something is natural doesn't mean it can't be harmful, especially when combined with other treatments. As an example, ginkgo, an extract made from the seeds and leaves of the Chinese ginkgo biloba tree, is sometimes used to improve thinking and memory in healthy people as well as those with dementia. However, it should not be combined with certain drugs, for instance blood-thinning drugs such as warfarin, or with anti-depressants.

As well as checking the credentials of any complementary practitioner you see, you should also let the medical professionals caring for you or your loved one know that you are thinking of trying complementary therapies, and tell them about any treatments and medication you are prescribed by anyone else.

Both the Alzheimer's Society and the Royal College of Psychiatrists (contact details on pp. 107 and 110) have a lot of useful information about the value of different complementary treatments for all kinds of dementia. It's interesting to remember that Reminyl, one of the three main licensed medicines for the treatment of Alzheimer's, was originally derived from snowdrop and narcissi bulbs, so could be said to be a herbal preparation itself.

What kinds of complementary medicine might help someone with dementia?

Herbal medicine

Herbal remedies are made from plants, and at one time all medicine was herbal medicine. Many modern drugs – not just Reminyl – were originally derived from plant sources, for example aspirin and some anti-cancer drugs. In Britain, herbal remedies are obtainable over the counter from pharmacies and health food shops. For a more detailed and personal treatment plan, it's advisable to consult a qualified medical herbalist. Always look for 'standardized' herbal remedies – in other words, those where the amount of active ingredient will be the same in every tablet or bottle. Some of the herbs which have been used to improve memory and concentration include:

- ginkgo
- ginseng
- sage
- lemon balm.

As yet, researchers don't seem to know quite how any of these herbal remedies work, and the evidence that they can actually help, though interesting, is not overwhelming. Ginkgo, for example, may have anti-oxidant qualities which prevent cell damage, and may increase the blood flow or chemical transmitters within the brain. Like all medication it can cause side effects, as mentioned above. Ginseng, which is grown in many parts of the world, could work by thinning the blood, or, like ginkgo, have anti-oxidant qualities. It should not be combined with anti-diabetes drugs, blood-thinning agents or some anti-depressants. Sage – which has had a reputation for ensuring a long and healthy life since ancient times – has also been used to improve memory and concentration and may have anti-oxidant qualities as well as increasing some of the chemical transmitters in the brain.

There is some evidence that lemon balm has a calming effect and it has been used to treat agitation in people with dementia. The Mental Health Foundation funded some research at Newcastle University in 2000 which discovered that lemon balm could do more than simply help to relax and calm people with dementia. In addition, it seemed to help prevent the loss of the brain chemical acetylcholine in the same way as the first two anti-Alzheimer's drugs, Aricept and Exelon.

Other herbs, such as lavender and valerian, can have a calming and relaxing effect and are sometimes prescribed by herbalists to help with sleep problems.

Traditional Chinese medicine

Traditional Chinese medicine (TCM) works on completely different principles from those we are familiar with in the West. The principle is that all ill health is caused by an imbalance in the correct flow of the life-force, known as *Qi* or *Chi*, through the twelve pathways or meridians, six of which are Yin (feminine, cold, passive) and six Yang (masculine, hot, active.) The aim of Chinese medicine is to balance these elements, resulting in good health.

Chinese medicine is based on syndromes, not just symptoms, and if you consult a Chinese doctor you will be asked about all aspects of your general health. Your tongue will be examined and your pulse taken before any treatment is suggested. The best-known treatments in TCM are acupuncture and Chinese herbs. According to the Alzheimer's Society, there have been a few studies suggesting that acupuncture – which attempts to unblock the meridians by the use of very fine needles – can improve cognitive functioning as well as alleviate anxiety and depression.

Herbal preparations have been studied in both China and Japan, where some are used to treat dementia. A chemical called Huperzine A, made from the plant *Huperzia serrata*, has been found to improve memory in people with Alzheimer's and vascular dementia. The practice of Chinese herbal medicine in Japan, known as *kanpo*, is integrated into the Japanese health-care system. Some of the herbal mixtures used appear to help slow the decline in cognitive function. More research is needed on these.

Nutrition therapy

Nutrition therapy is 'on the borders' of complementary medicine. It's generally agreed that eating a healthy balanced diet including some foods from all food groups will benefit people with early-onset Alzheimer's, as it does everyone else. However, there are nutritionists who claim that particular foods or supplements can also be beneficial, and there is some evidence that this may be true.

Anti-oxidant compounds, which are mostly found in fruit and vegetables, may help to prevent conditions such as Alzheimer's as well as other serious diseases. They are substances which prevent cell damage by 'free radicals' – the kind of damage which causes peeled apples to turn brown, metals to rust, and oils to become rancid. High daily doses of Vitamin E, which is found in wheatgerm and sunflower seed oils, nuts, seeds, avocados and spinach, were found in one study to help prevent falls in those with Alzheimer's. Two other anti-oxidants, selegiline, which is already used in the treatment of Parkinson's disease, and idebenone, which seems to help by increasing the production of vital brain chemicals, are also being studied and both seem to have positive effects.

B vitamins have also been recommended as a way of preventing and/or slowing down the progress of dementia. A diet rich in folic acid, found in leafy green vegetables, has been suggested as a way of helping to repair damage to nerve cells in some areas of the brain. American researchers have found that folic acid and Vitamin B12 lower the levels of an amino-acid in the blood which is often raised in people with Alzheimer's. An Oxford University study published in September 2010 found that Vitamin B supplements could slow down the rate of brain atrophy in older people with mild cognitive impairment. Vitamin B1 – otherwise known as thiamine – is needed for the glucose in the blood to produce the essential neurotransmitter acetylcholine. Thiamine is found in fortified breakfast cereals, wholemeal bread and pasta, yeast extract, peas, oranges and eggs, and has been shown to improve both memory and concentration.

Another substance which has anti-oxidant properties and has been used to treat dementia is bee propolis. This is a resinous substance which is gathered by bees from the buds and bark of trees and other types of vegetation, mixed with their own secretions, and may be used to 'disinfect' the hive and protect the eggs. It is already known that propolis has healing, anti-microbial and anti-inflammatory properties, and more trials are needed to discover whether it is really useful as a treatment, and how it might work.

Aromatherapy and massage

Aromatherapy is the use of essential oils derived from plants for therapeutic purposes. These oils may be massaged directly into the skin, heated in an oil burner or added to a bath. According to the Alzheimer's Society, the combination of the right essential oils and massage can be effective in reducing anxiety and agitation and 'wandering'. There are many different types of massage and anyone interested in exploring this form of therapy should contact the General Council for Massage Therapies (contact details on p. 109). More large-scale trials are needed of different types of massage, different aromatherapy oils and different forms of dementia.

Music and art therapy

Sessions with a specially trained music or art therapist can also improve the quality of life for some people with dementia and their families and carers. As is the case with most complementary treatments, there is little published, high-quality research to 'prove' the therapeutic value of this kind of therapy. However, music and art therapists are increasingly working with people with dementia and report that exposure to both art and music – either creating music or artwork themselves, or listening to music or looking at painting or sculpture – can result in better moods, more interaction with other people, and a reduction in challenging behaviour. Strangely, it is also reported that some people with fronto-temporal dementia actually develop an aptitude for art.

Melatonin and 'bright light' therapy

Many people with early-onset dementia suffer from sleep disturbances, and caring for someone who gets up and wanders at night is one of the most exhausting aspects of being a carer. 'Sundowning', when the person is especially restless and agitated in the late afternoon and early evening, is a recognized phenomenon.

In some research studies, people who had sleeping problems were treated with the hormone melatonin, which is known to be involved in the normal cycle of sleeping and waking. (It is also sometimes advocated as a cure for jet lag.) Melatonin, which is released by a small gland in the centre of the brain called the pineal gland, is suppressed by light and stimulated by darkness. Normal sleeping and waking cycles in humans seem to be disturbed by dementia.

Wakeful behaviour during the night was treated in one study by a combination of melatonin and 'bright light' therapy, which did seem to calm the restless behaviour. Again, further research would seem to be needed on this.

What kinds of complementary therapies might help carers and families?

Most complementary therapists are trained to look at people 'holistically' – that is, they look at the whole person, not just one particular symptom. Anyone caring for a loved one with early-onset dementia is likely to be feeling tired, stressed, sad, angry and/or frustrated – part of the time or, indeed, most of the time. In Chapter 7 we have already touched on the importance of 'caring for the carers' and complementary therapies may have a part to play in that. Relaxation and stress reduction are among the results promised by many of these therapies. Carers might particularly benefit from relaxation therapies such as yoga, meditation and autogenic training (AT).

Yoga, for example, has been developed over thousands of years to promote good physical health and inner peace. The roots of yoga go back to the dawn of Indian civilization – the word 'yoga' is derived from a Sanskrit word meaning 'union'. Yoga helps to promote union between mind and body by the use of correct breathing and physical exercises. Gentle stretching and breathing improve peace of mind and help to maintain the flow of energy. Yoga can help to control and still the mind and reduce stress. It is non-competitive, you do not have to be a contortionist, and the best way to benefit is to join a class. The British Wheel of Yoga (contact details on p. 108) can give information about classes in your area.

Different kinds of meditation – transcendental meditation and Buddhist meditation among them – can help people who practise them to achieve a state of deep and complete relaxation. Once you have learned how to meditate, a 20-minute session twice a day can benefit your physical, mental and emotional health and help to combat stress and anxiety. EEGs (electroencephalograms) have shown that meditation produces alpha-waves in the brain which are associated with rest and relaxation. T'ai chi, sometimes known as 'meditation in motion', combines gentle exercise with meditation and is often recommended for those suffering from stress.

Autogenic training was devised by a German doctor back in the 1920s. AT is rather similar to meditation and self-hypnosis. An autogenic training course teaches you a series of very simple, repetitive instructions which are designed to promote deep relaxation and switch off the 'fight or flight' response which leads to so much stress and tension. Introduced into Britain in the 1970s, AT has been shown to help stress-related conditions and improve the quality of sleep.

Massage is probably the earliest form of therapy known to humankind. Practised in many different styles and different cultures, it involves a trained massage therapist soothing the knots out of tense muscles using various different touching techniques. Stroking, pummelling, tapping, knuckling and wringing may all be used, with or without the addition of calming essential oils.

Bach flower remedies were devised by a Harley Street physician and homoeopath, Dr Edward Bach, to treat negative or harmful states of mind. There are 38 of them, and you are advised to match them to your own mood, situation or personality. You can mix up to seven remedies together if it seems appropriate. Bach practitioner Nishma says that the remedy impatiens could help carers who are impatient with others' slowness. Walnut is appropriate at times of great change, for example when you see the first signs of dementia in someone you love. Elm should be chosen if you feel overwhelmed by your many responsibilities. For more information, you could consult a registered Bach Foundation practitioner or contact the Bach Centre in Oxfordshire – contact details on p. 107.

9

Caring in the later stages

According to the Alzheimer's Society, about a third of the people who have dementia are in residential care. Even though a partner or carer's instinctive reaction, on learning of a relative's diagnosis, may well be 'I could never put you in a home!' most people with early-onset dementia do eventually need to be in residential care.

The whole question of long-term care for the mentally infirm is something that politicians, clinicians, carers and those with dementia themselves argue about, and there is no one 'right answer' for every case. Would it really be better if everyone in the later stages of this distressing condition could be cared for at home, with support from Social Services? Too often, 'care in the community' has come to mean everything being landed on families. The image of residential care or nursing homes is of elderly people slumped in armchairs while a TV screen blares, unwatched, in the centre of the room. It's no wonder that many families feel guilty if they find themselves even considering a residential placement for a loved one.

Specialist provision for people with early-onset dementia is still not widely available, though there is a growing awareness that the care needs of this group *are* different from those of much older people. The best residential homes which do specialize in the care of those with early-onset dementia can be very good indeed. Families also worry about who is going to pay for long-term, high-quality care, much of which is provided by private companies. It's reassuring to know that even in private care homes, some state help with funding is often available.

BUPA, for instance, say that two-thirds of the residents in their care homes get some financial assistance from the National Health Service or Social Services. PJ Care, the company which runs Bluebirds, a care home for those with early-onset dementia in Milton Keynes, say that most of their residents are funded by their primary care trust as there is nowhere else suitable for them to live.

Home care

Some people are, of course, able to be cared for at home even when their condition has progressed to its later stages. Much depends on their symptoms and how difficult management becomes, as well as on the carer or carers and their other commitments. When a carer's circumstances change – for instance, if he or she becomes ill or can no longer offer appropriate care – or the condition of the person with dementia deteriorates, Social Services should be asked for a reassessment. It is always possible that extra home care could be provided, perhaps in the form of extra time at the day centre, or help from the Crossroads Care Attendance Scheme, Admiral nurses or your local community psychiatric nurse. If you want, and are able, to buy in private care at home, the organization to contact is the United Kingdom Homecare Association (contact details on p. 111), who have information about the companies providing home care. Like care homes, companies providing care in people's own homes are inspected by the Care Quality Commission (contact details on p. 108), whose website has useful information about what to look for.

Top-quality home care should be flexible. Carers should be able to fit in with your schedule and habits, not expect you to fit in with theirs at all times. It's good practice for them to ask you – and the person with dementia, if appropriate – what needs to be done and when, and also for the same carers to become regulars, so that both the person with dementia and the family can get to know them. Poor practice includes employing carers who are too rushed to chat and get to know the people they are caring for, who don't speak adequate English, and who have too rigid a timetable, so that they might not arrive to help the person out of bed until lunch time, or are ready to put someone to bed in the early evening.

Thinking about residential care

The decision to look for residential care for a loved one, whatever that person's condition, is always going to be difficult. Many people and families affected by early-onset dementia say that they prefer to live from day to day, without thinking too much about what the future may hold. This is understandable, but on the other hand planning ahead can be useful so that when the person with dementia becomes ill enough for residential care to be considered, families and carers have some idea of what his or her wishes are. Many carers are forced to look for residential care when there has been some kind of crisis in the family, and in those circumstances choices are bound to be more limited. How do you know when the time is right? Is it really best for everyone? What does the person him or herself actually feel about it? How can you be sure the home you choose is somewhere your loved one will be happy and have as good a quality of life as possible?

Chris Ardill of the Relatives' and Residents' Association, a group campaigning for the rights of people in care, says:

> There is less suitable accommodation available for people with early-onset dementia than there is for older people, or people with learning difficulties. More awareness of dementia does mean that some care homes are beginning to offer specialized facilities for younger people. As an example there is the Old Deanery in Essex [contact details on p. 110] which has 190 beds for EOD [early-onset dementia] people in a 'care village' with special facilities like art and craft classes, physio- and occupational therapy and complementary therapies.

Chris is frequently contacted by family members thinking about residential care for their loved ones, many of whom need to be reassured that they are doing the right thing. He comments:

> People so often feel they have failed when relatives have to go into care. But the idea that everyone is better off in their own home means nothing. Old or sick people can be virtual prisoners in their own homes; isolated, without activities or stimulation. Families may be able to cope with a condition like dementia in its early stages, but later the level of care required could be beyond their skills, no matter how much they love the person who is ill. They may not be able to lift them or keep them properly clean, especially if they have other commitments such as jobs and children to look after. The best care homes can cope with difficult behaviour, such as wandering, by providing a high level of staffing or an enclosed garden where someone with dementia who wanders is quite safe.
>
> Medical professionals, Social Services, the library, the town hall, carers' support groups, an organization called Care Choices [contact details on p. 108] and the Internet are all good sources of information about the residential care that is available.

The charity Sue Ryder Care (contact details on p. 110) provides care services to people with long-term care needs. As well as providing home care, it has seven residential centres for people with neurological conditions such as Huntington's, Parkinson's and motor neurone disease, as well as dementia.

Nancy's husband Geoff, who had frontal lobe dementia, was cared for at home for four years before Nancy made the difficult decision to look for a residential place for him.

> I had to carry on working as I had a mortgage to pay. Our Social Services sent carers round to help with Geoff's personal care and he went on bus trips to clubs, but most of the other people there were 80-plus and the activities provided weren't right for him, although he did enjoy going.
>
> The Clive Project was our lifeline. Someone came round twice a week to be with Geoff, went for walks with him and encouraged his interest in photography. But eventually, full-time care seemed the only option. We had two deluges when he turned taps on and flooded the house. He walked and counted and paced continually, including going out and

pacing round complete strangers' gardens, which of course upset them. He also went out at night and locked himself out. We began looking for a residential place, and although the one we eventually chose didn't have particular experience of early-onset dementia they were fantastic.

Of course it was sad at first. Geoff even said, 'I'm being evicted from this family!' which was heartbreaking. But once he was settled in with a plate of macaroni cheese and a glass of wine, he said 'Cheers!' as I left. Geoff had previously been a social worker and the staff of the care home let him sit in the office and arrange the files, which helped him to keep his dignity. It was a real family atmosphere.

Choosing a care home

The Alzheimer's Society says that the ideal care home is one which preserves dignity, treats residents with respect, promotes independence and provides a good quality of life. This is true whether the person concerned has early-onset dementia or any other condition. The concept of 'person-centred care' – which is provided in the best care homes – was pioneered by Professor Tom Kitwood back in the 1990s. In his book *Dementia Reconsidered: The person comes first* (Open University Press, 1997), he challenged old ideas and tried to understand what 'being in care' was like from the point of view of the person with dementia.

'Person-centred care' is all about treating residents the way you would like to be treated yourself, focusing on the person as an individual, not on the illness. Understanding and well-trained care staff realize that challenging behaviour may be an attempt to communicate, and use various kinds of stimuli, including non-verbal stimuli, to communicate with residents. Nor do they let residents think that the things they say are stupid or irrelevant. Every resident is a human being, with a history, likes and dislikes, habits and pleasures, and should be treated as though he or she matters.

How can carers and families ensure that the residential care they choose comes up to those high standards? The first thing to do is to find out whether there are care homes in your area which make special provision for people with early-onset dementia. If there is nothing local, it might be possible to obtain funding for a more suitable placement in a different area, if that would better meet the person's needs (for more on funding, see pp. 101–3). As well as those already mentioned, the Priory Group runs ten specialist 'complex care' hospitals, Hillcroft Nursing Homes have specialist units for people with early-onset dementia and Barchester Care Homes are among the other companies who can provide some specialist facilities.

You will want to visit several homes before making your choice. These days the distinction between 'residential homes', which provide personal care such as help with washing, dressing and feeding, and 'nursing homes', where there has to be a qualified nurse on duty at all times, has been changed slightly. All are now referred to as 'registered care homes', but in addition are described as '*with* nursing' or '*with* dementia care'. Not everyone with dementia needs nursing care, and the nurses on duty in some care homes may not be mental-health nurses.

What should you look for? Many privately run homes send out a glossy brochure, but there's no substitute for a visit and a chat to staff, managers, residents and residents' families. Remember that this place may eventually be your relative's home, so a warm, homely, welcoming atmosphere is very important. It goes without saying that it should be clean, and the location should be appropriate, with access to the local community if possible and transport for outings. Residents should, as far as possible, seem responsive, happy, dressed, alert, talkative and engaged with other residents and staff in conversation or activities.

What are the rooms like? Can residents bring their own furniture, personal possessions, pets? Is their privacy respected? Are issues like incontinence tactfully dealt with, and are there enough toilets within easy reach of bedrooms and lounges?

Is there somewhere quiet where residents can meet their families? Do they have access to a garden? Are visitors welcome, including children? What sort of activities are arranged? Is there a choice of food at mealtimes? Are residents helped to eat if necessary? Can they make drinks and snacks for themselves if they want to?

You know your relative best – is this the kind of place he or she could settle and feel at home? Is there scope for any hobbies or interests that could be maintained, such as gardening? Could individual requests like that be accommodated?

Staff should be warm, friendly and caring, with time to chat and get to know residents, and the manager should be welcoming, experienced in the care of people with early-onset dementia, and able to treat each resident as an individual with individual tastes, needs and problems.

It sounds like a tall order, but the best care homes try to be all those things, as explained by Lyn Meehan, research and development nurse from PJ Care, the company which runs Bluebirds in Milton Keynes.

> Bluebirds, which specializes in the care of early-onset dementia, has been open for some time, and was designed to be a therapeutic environment. So many people with early-onset dementia end up in homes designed for much older people where their specific needs may not be met.
>
> Our residents have individual therapy, are able to move around freely and have their behaviour supported. We only use medication to control challenging behaviour in an emergency and all care is very much person-centred and one-to-one. Bluebirds has beautiful gardens for residents to enjoy, where they are quite safe but not 'locked in'. We have a minibus for outings and an activities support team, with all activities tailored to the individual and covering things like cookery, table tennis, cultural days – whatever is appropriate and enjoyable.
>
> Most of our residents have frontal or temporal lobe dementias or conditions like Huntington's and they are mostly in their fifties. They usually come to us after a breakdown in family care.

They can be with us for six to eight years or longer and we offer strong end-of-life care, which helps the relatives as well as the residents. There is an active relatives' group as well. We take referrals from all over the UK.

Jean had to go outside her local area to find appropriate care for her brother, who was diagnosed with a rare form of vascular dementia when he was just 40.

Our county is a 'black hole' as far as residential care is concerned. They only cater for very elderly people and the quality is not that good. Eventually I found somewhere excellent for David. Even though it is 50 miles away, I knew it was the right home for him. I have total faith in the person who runs it. She really *listens*, both to residents and their families. David's first room was very noisy as several of the residents nearby wandered around and screamed and shouted, so David was moved to another wing which is quieter. He also has a double bed in his room, which the manager agreed was part of being an adult!

David can come and go as he pleases. We have an account with a local taxi firm which comes to take him to the bookshop and café in the nearest town so he still feels in control of his life. He has a regular visitor from the Clive Project who takes him out and plays chess with him. I went with him to join the library.

Occasionally there are problems – for instance, I had to persuade them to send him to the dentist! His speech has deteriorated a lot and he was finding it hard and frustrating trying to make himself understood to some of the staff who were foreign-born. He was angry and resentful at first that he had to go into care, but after a settling-in period, he seems happy. Some facets of his brain and personality are still there and he can stay until he dies.

I would advise families to start looking at residential care homes before you really need to. It's only by going and looking at what is available that you begin to understand what is needed. There are things you might not think of. For example, I soon realized David would not be happy if he was in the depths of the country. He needed to be part of the community so that he could make the most of the facilities available, like the library and the coffee shop, where everyone now knows him. Somewhere with gloomy, depressing views from the windows, or somewhere dominated by the TV, wouldn't have been right for him either.

I also think it helps if a person goes into care while they still have enough of their faculties to be able to bond with the staff and possibly the other residents, and while their personality still shows through. There is appropriate care out there; it's just a question of finding it.

Legal issues

It is not easy to balance the legal rights of those with early-onset dementia and their carers with the 'duty of care' placed on local authorities, who are legally obliged to care for vulnerable adults in their area. The Mental Capacity Act 2005 states that people should be supported in making decisions for themselves if they are capable of doing so, and that decisions should be made 'in their best interests' if they are too mentally infirm to make their own. Any assessment or care plan by health or Social Services should meet the needs of the person with dementia and the local authority should always act 'in their best interests'.

This can cover situations such as people being unwilling to go into residential care, carers stating they are no longer able to care for someone, or local authorities wanting to place someone in a home which families believe does not meet their needs. Both people with dementia and their carers have rights in these situations, and if you're faced with a dilemma of this kind you can obtain advice from the Alzheimer's Society and the other support groups for people with early-onset dementia. The principle that anyone needing residential care should only be placed in a care home which meets his or her individual needs is an important one and if you don't feel your relative is getting a fair deal you are entitled to appeal.

Paying for care

The rules about who pays for what in the funding of long-term care are complex and continually argued over by politicians of all parties. Very broadly speaking, it will depend on:

- the type of care required – at present in England and Wales but not Scotland, 'nursing' care is paid for by the state – the NHS in fact – but 'personal' care is not; and

- the person's financial circumstances – income, benefits, savings, and so on.

Local Social Services are responsible for arranging funding for vulnerable adults assessed as needing to be in a care home. They may pay all or part of the cost of care, depending on the person's means. Other people, known as 'self-funders', arrange and pay for their own care, but if you plan – and can afford – to do this you should obtain a Social Services assessment anyway, in case your circumstances change in the future. Self-funders are entitled to claim benefits to help with care home fees. As we have seen, many of those in privately run care homes have their fees paid wholly or partly by their local authorities. Nursing care is free and funded by the NHS.

Once someone has been assessed as needing to be in a care home, Social Services will do a financial assessment in order to work out how much that person must contribute towards his or her own care. This assessment will look closely at the family's circumstances, taking into account both income, including income from state benefits, and capital, including savings, investments and the value of the family home.

Exactly how much an individual will have to contribute to his or her own care varies from year to year and from local authority to local authority. You will be expected to claim all the benefits you are entitled to, in order to help pay care home fees. Some benefits do not count as income.

Local authorities all have 'price limits', but set against the financial considerations is the principle that those assessed as needing care should be accommodated somewhere that 'meets their needs'. This could mean that a more expensive but more suitable care home could be funded by a particular local authority. All the person's needs – including the need to be near family or friends – must be taken into account. Local authorities may also agree to pay for a more expensive care home if someone else pays 'top-up' fees – for instance family or a charity. (See pp. 61 and 107–11 for information about charities which can offer financial help for people in these circumstances.)

You do not have to sell your home to pay for care if it is occupied by the person's wife, husband, partner, a relative under 16 or over 60, or a disabled relative under 60.

You are always entitled to appeal if you are not happy with the arrangements made by the NHS or Social Services.

End-of-life care

End-of-life care – or 'palliative care' as it is sometimes known – can be provided at home, in care homes, in hospitals and hospices. The charity Sue Ryder Care (contact details on p. 110) is one of the largest providers of specialist palliative care in the UK in its six specialist hospices. Local palliative care teams look after not only the person but also the family at this difficult time. Specially trained nurses can take care of the person's physical well-being, making sure that immobility doesn't lead to pressure sores, for instance, and also that the medication prescribed is appropriate and helps that person to be as comfortable as possible. Once he or she can no longer recognize those around, or communicate, it can be comforting simply to hold hands, stroke the person gently, perhaps talk to him or her, play some much-loved music or burn some scented oils.

In the case of someone with dementia, difficult decisions have to be made about how long life should be prolonged in these circumstances. This is why it can be helpful, at an earlier stage, for the family to discuss what the person's wishes are. The Alzheimer's Society has information about 'advance decisions', otherwise known as Living Wills or Advance Directives, which allow people to set out their wishes in writing.

Life expectancy for people with early-onset dementia varies and tends to be shorter than for those diagnosed later in life. Very sick people are vulnerable to infections such as pneumonia; they may have heart conditions or simply stop eating. At this point families and medical professionals will have to discuss the options and make a decision based on the person's own wishes or, if these are not known, in that person's best interests.

Cathy was diagnosed with early-onset Alzheimer's five years ago, when she was in her late forties. Since then she has been taking Aricept, which has enabled her to live a near-normal life and has also given her time to discuss the future with her husband and grown-up children.

> My grandmother had dementia, and so did my father, and having seen their later years, I have made my plans with my husband. Although he finds it very difficult to talk about, or even think about, I have told him that when I get to the point that I don't know my family any longer, I don't want to be given any more medication. I hope that will end my life more quickly.
>
> I want my family to have happy memories of me, unlike the memories I have of my gran, who didn't know any of us for years and was 101 when she died. In the final stages of dementia, I will no longer be 'me'. I will just be a shell. Everything that makes me 'me' will have gone. I don't want to live like that, for my own sake as well as the sake of my family.
>
> It is sad that many people with dementia don't get a diagnosis until it's too late for them to make their wishes known.

Coping with bereavement

We have already seen in Chapter 7 that grief and a sense of loss are very much part of the experience of caring for someone with early-onset dementia. Partners and families begin the grieving process while the person they love is still alive. You are grieving for the person you knew, the relationship you once had, the life you once had, the plans you made together. Another milestone is passed when the person with dementia has to go into residential care. Even when you know it was the best decision there will still be a sense of loss, and often guilt as well.

Losing a loved partner is the worst thing that can happen to any of us. It's the price we pay for loving and there is no 'right way' to deal with it. You may feel completely numb at first – or a confusing mixture of emotions ranging from sadness, anger or bitterness to relief that your loved one's suffering is over and a huge sense of loss because this illness, which has dominated all your lives for so long, has now done its worst.

Now is the time to look after yourself. Take it a day at a time, without thinking too much about the future. You have spent so long caring for another person, in every sense of the word – now you need to take care of *you*. Accept all the help that you are offered, from friends, family, your GP, the palliative care team, the staff at the care home, the support groups for those with early-onset dementia.

Above all, remember that everything you are feeling is natural and that no-one can, or should try to, tell you that you 'should' feel this, or do that. We all grieve in our own way and in our own time. Cruse Bereavement Care (contact details on p. 108) are the experts in caring for those who have been bereaved and can offer help and information about bereavement counselling.

Nancy's husband Geoff died suddenly in his care home in 2009.

> The care he received could not have been better. He was given morphine and made comfortable and the family were able to be with him until the end.
>
> When he died, it was easier for me in a way because I had already lost the Geoff I knew. In his final years we had more of a mother–child relationship. I was there to make sure everything went well for him. I had already done some of my grieving. I was glad the end came quickly. Some of the care home residents were lying on sheepskins, just being fed and having their hands held, and I didn't want that for Geoff. Now,

when the children and I think and talk about him, we remember him as he was before he was ill.

It's said that bereavement progresses in stages – from shock and denial, through sadness, to eventual acceptance. You may go through some or all of those stages, or you may not, and there is no timetable. Grief is not a linear process but more of a roller-coaster. You can think you are dealing with it all quite well until something – often a quite minor incident – reminds you and sends you back to the beginning again. But you never do go right back to the beginning. If you can talk about the person you loved, share the feelings, both happy and sad, and the memories, with others who loved him or her, acceptance will come and life can – and will – go on.

Useful addresses

ABF The Soldiers' Charity: tel.: 0845 241 4820; website: www.soldierscharity.org

AcuMedic (Chinese medical centre): tel.: 020 7388 6704; website: www.acumedic.com

Admiral Nursing DIRECT: tel.: 0845 257 9406 (helpline staffed by Admiral nurses trained in dementia care; 11 a.m. to 8.45 p.m., Tuesday and Thursday; 10 a.m. to 1 p.m., Saturday); website: www.dementiauk.org

Age UK: tel.: 0800 169 6565 (advice line); website: www.ageuk.org.uk; offers information on all aspects of life for older people

Alzheimer's Research Trust: tel.: 01223 843899; website: www.alzheimers-research.org.uk

Alzheimer's Society: National Dementia Helpline: 0845 300 0336 (8.30 a.m. to 6.30 p.m., Monday to Friday); website: www.alzheimers.org.uk

AT Dementia: tel.: 0116 257 5017; website: www.atdementia.org.uk; for information on assistive technology for people with dementia

Bach Centre: tel.: 01491 832 877 (consultation line); website: www.bachcentre.com; for Bach flower remedies

Barchester Care Homes: tel.: 020 7352 2224; website: www.barchester. com; runs care homes all over the UK, some with special provision for people with early-onset dementia

Bladder and Bowel Foundation: tel.: 01536 533255 (general enquiries); 0845 345 0165 (specialist Continence Nurse helpline for medical advice); website: www.bladderandbowelfoundation.org; for help with incontinence

Brain and Spine Foundation: tel.: 0808 808 1000 (helpline); website: www.brainandspine.org.uk

British Acupuncture Council: tel.: 020 8735 0400; website: www.acupuncture.org.uk

British Association of Art Therapists: tel.: 0207 686 4216; website: www.baat.org

British Association for Counselling and Psychotherapy: tel.: 01455 883300; website: www.bacp.org.uk

British Autogenic Society: tel.: 0207 391 8908; website: www.autogenic-therapy.org.uk

British Society for Music Therapy: tel.: 0207 837 6100; website: www.bsmt.org

British Wheel of Yoga: tel.: 01529 306851; website: www.bwy.org.uk

Care Choices: tel.: 01223 207770; website: www.carechoices.co.uk; for information about available care options

Care Quality Commission: tel.: 03000 616161 (8.30 a.m. to 5.30 p.m., Monday to Friday); website: www.cqc.org.uk; offers advice on choosing social care

Carers UK: tel.: 0808 808 7777 (advice line; 10 a.m. to 12 noon and 2 p.m. to 4 p.m., Wednesday and Thursday); website: www.carersuk.org

Citizens Advice: tel.: 020 7833 2181 (admin only); website: www. citizensadvice.org.uk

CJD Support Network: tel.: 01630 673993 (admin); 01630 673973 (helpline); website: www.cjdsupport.net

Clive Project: tel.: 01993 776295; website: www.thecliveproject.org.uk; Oxfordshire-based support group for people with early-onset dementia and their families

Crossroads Care (England and Wales): tel.: 0845 450 0350 (office); website: www.crossroads.org.uk

Crossroads Caring for Carers (Northern Ireland): tel.: 028 9181 4455; website: www.crossroadscare.co.uk

Crossroads Caring Scotland: tel.: 0141 226 3793; website: www.crossroads-scotland.co.uk

Cruse Bereavement Care: tel.: 020 8939 9530; daytime helpline: 0844 477 9400; website: www.crusebereavementcare.org.uk

Dementia UK: tel.: 0207 874 7200; website: www.dementiauk.org; dedicated to improving the quality of life for people with dementia

Disabled Living Foundation: tel.: 020 7289 6111; helpline: 0845 130 9177 (10 a.m. to 4 p.m., Monday to Friday); website: www.dlf. org.uk; offers advice on equipment to help those with special needs

Down's Syndrome Association: tel.: 0845 230 0372 (helpline; 10 a.m. to 4 p.m., Monday to Friday); website: www.downs-syndrome.org.uk

Driver and Vehicle Licensing Agency (DVLA): tel.: 0300 790 6801 (drivers' enquiries); 0300 790 6806 (medical enquiries); website: www.dft.gov.uk/dvla/

Elizabeth Finn Care: tel.: 020 8834 9200; website: www.elizabethfinncare. org.uk; provides grants for families in need

Enable Holidays: tel.: 0871 222 4939; website: www.enableholidays.com; offers information about holidays in Europe and the USA for people with special needs

Equality and Human Rights Commission: tel. (helpline): 0845 604 6610 (England); 0845 604 5510 (Scotland); 0845 604 8810 (Wales); website: www.equalityhumanrights.com

General Council for Massage Therapies: tel.: 0870 850 4452; website: www.gcmt.org.uk

Hearing and Mobility: tel.: 0844 888 1338; website: www. hearingandmobility.co.uk; sells aids to daily living including mobility and incontinence aids

Hillcroft Nursing Homes: tel.: 01524 734433; website: www. hillcroftnursinghomes.co.uk; runs care homes in north-west England

Huntington's Disease Association (HDA): tel.: 0151 298 3298; website: www.hda.org.uk

International Federation of Aromatherapists: tel.: 0208 567 2243; website: www.ifaroma.org

Law Society: tel.: 020 7242 1222; website: www.lawsociety.org.uk

MedicAlert: tel.: 0800 581420 (freephone); website: www.medicalert.org.uk; supplies jewellery that identifies people with medical problems

Mental Health Foundation: tel.: 020 7803 1101 (to order publications); 020 7803 1100 (to find out about the organization's work); website: www.mentalhealth.org.uk; has information on mental-health issues but does not run a helpline

Motor Neurone Disease (MND) Association: tel.: 01604 250505; MND Connect: 08457 626262 (advice, practical and emotional support and directing to other services and agencies); website: www.mndassociation.org

Multiple Sclerosis Society: tel.: 0808 800 8000 (freephone helpline); website: www.mssociety.org.uk

National Debtline: tel.: 0808 808 4000 (helpline; 9 a.m. to 9 p.m., Monday to Friday; 9.30 a.m. to 1 p.m., Saturday); website: www. nationaldebtline.co.uk

National Institute of Medical Herbalists: tel.: 01392 426022; website: www.nimh.org.uk

Natural Death Centre: tel.: 01962 712690 (helpline); website: www.naturaldeath.org.uk; provides information on Advance Directives or Living Wills

NHS Free Smoking Helpline: tel.: 0800 022 4332 (7 a.m. to 11 p.m., seven days a week); website: http://smokefree.nhs.uk

Office of the Public Guardian: tel.: 0300 456 0300; website: www.publicguardian.gov.uk; offers information about Powers of Attorney and the Court of Protection

Old Deanery: tel.: 01376 328600; website: www.olddeanery.com; care village with facilities for those with early-onset dementia

Parkinson's UK: tel.: 0808 800 0303 (helpline); website: www.parkinsons.org.uk

Pick's Disease Support Group: tel.: 01297 445488; website: www.pdsg.org.uk

PJ Care: tel.: 01908 634995; website: www.pjcare.co.uk; runs care homes for people with early-onset dementia

Princess Royal Trust for Carers: tel.: 0844 800 4361; website: www.carers.org

Priory Group: tel.: 0845 277 4679; website: www.priorygroup.com; independent provider of care homes

RAF Benevolent Fund: tel.: 0800 169 2942 (support line); website: www.rafbf.org

Relate: tel.: 0300 100 1234; website: www.relate.org.uk; helps with all relationship problems

Relatives' and Residents' Association: tel.: 020 7359 8136 (advice line; 9.30 a.m. to 4.30 p.m., Monday to Friday); website: www.relres.org; provides support with and information about going into residential care

Royal College of Psychiatrists: tel.: 0207 235 2351; website: www.rcpsych.ac.uk; produces leaflets on mental-health issues including dementia

Samaritans: tel.: 08457 909090; website: www.samaritans.org

SSAFA Forces Help: tel.: 0845 1300 975; website: www.ssafa.org.uk; help for serving and former military personnel and their families

Sue Ryder Care: tel.: 0845 050 1953; website: www.suerydercare.org

Sunrise Senior Living: tel.: 0800 012 1861; website: www.sunrise.care.co.uk; offers person-centred care, including for younger residents

Tourism for All: tel.: 0845 124 9971; website: www.tourismforall.org.uk; supplies information about holidays for those with special needs

Transcendental Meditation: tel.: 01695 51213; website: www.t-m.org.uk

United Kingdom Homecare Association: tel.: 020 8288 5291 (helpline); website: www.ukhca.co.uk

Vitalise: tel.: 0845 345 1970 (general enquiries); website: www.vitalise.org.uk; provides holiday centres for people with disabilities including dementia

Index